Adele Nozedar

THE GARDEN FORAGER

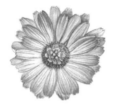

illustrated by Lizzie Harper

◧ SQUARE PEG

Adele's dedication
For Ty Neuadd

Lizzie's dedication
To my dear dad, John Harper, who taught me to love botany; and my lovely mum, Susan Harper, who taught me to love to draw.

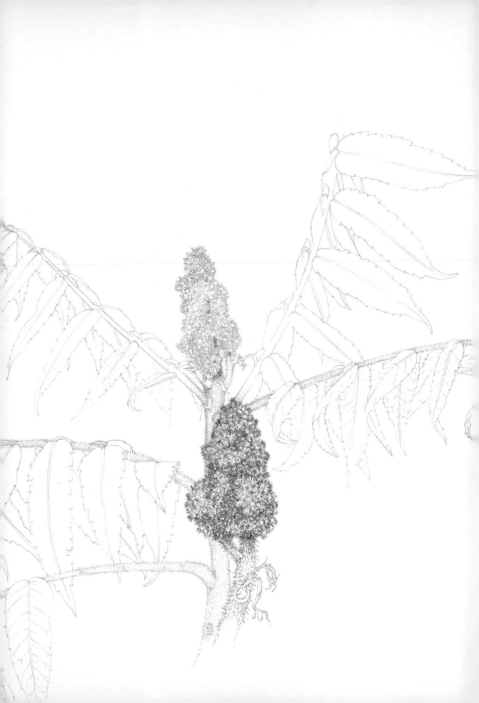

Putting in the Seed

Robert Frost

You come to fetch me from my work to-night
When supper's on the table, and we'll see
If I can leave off burying the white
Soft petals fallen from the apple tree
(Soft petals, yes, but not so barren quite,
Mingled with these, smooth bean and wrinkled pea;)
And go along with you ere you lose sight
Of what you came for and become like me,
Slave to a springtime passion for the earth.
How Love burns through the Putting in the Seed
On through the watching for that early birth
When, just as the soil tarnishes with weed,
The sturdy seedling with arched body comes
Shouldering its way and shedding the earth crumbs.

Contents

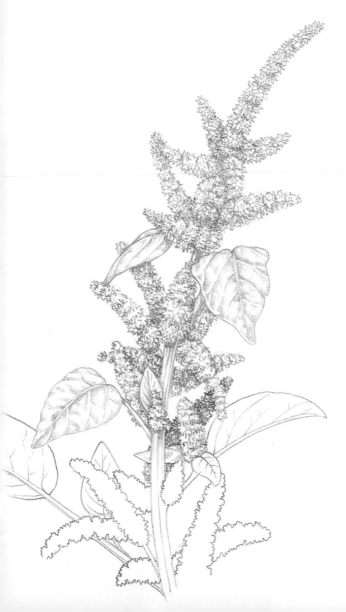

Introduction

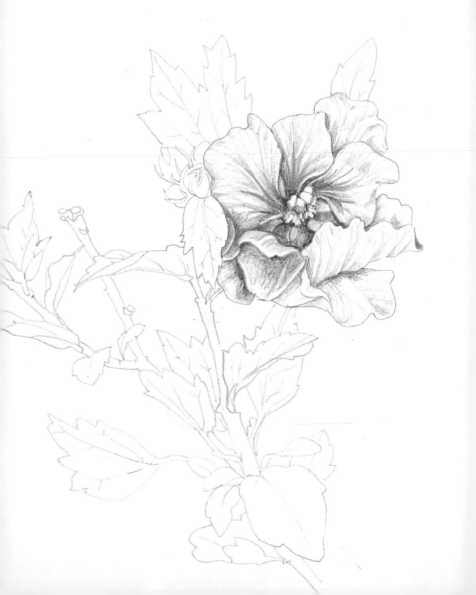

No fences in Eden

If you take a short drive out of Abergavenny into the rolling, folded hills of the old industrial part of South Wales around the small town of Blaenavon, you'll come to an amazing place, dubbed the Forgotten Landscapes. This is a designated UNESCO World Heritage site and therefore in the same league as more famous landmarks such as the Pyramids or the Great Wall of China. This particular stretch of the landscape is significant because the hidden hollows of these hills are the crucible in which the Industrial Revolution was founded. Around Blaenavon, the old iron works with their blast furnaces stand, still erect but derelict, bleak, disused, a humbling reminder that the works of mankind are barely a speck of dust in the greater picture. And growing out of a fissure in the side of a grim, tumbledown tram bridge is a lush, lavish, lovely but rather exotic (for this neck of the woods) fig tree.

How on earth did it get there? Did some homesick Italian immigrant, come to work in the furnaces over 200 years ago, sit on the bridge one day, legs dangling over the edge, forlornly eating the very last fig that he'd brought from Tuscany and thinking of the sunny home he'd never return to? Plants tell stories; this particular fig is a mute piece of living archaeology. We'll never know how it got there, but it's fun to try and guess.

Native to Western Asia and the Middle East, this sprawling fig tree couldn't have chosen many places quite so dissimilar to the arid dryness of its original sunny home. The higher hills of Wales are notorious for their weeks of snow, determined frosts and for the winds that whip the breath from your lungs and polish your nose and cheeks shiny red. Luckily, lots of the plants that have successfully spread themselves around the planet via various means – wind, water, the migrations of mammals and birds, even on the soles of our shoes – are extremely adaptable to alien habitats; jasmine, for example, which started out in the exotic East, but grows so well in Switzerland that plant collectors at one time thought that it must be indigenous to that country. Ah, plant collectors! Let's not forget the contribution these pioneers made, in helping plants to cross boundaries – political, cultural and horticultural.

Many of our common cultivated garden plants shared similarly exotic, exciting and adventurous pasts before they became part of our domestic landscape. It's also a bit of an eye-opener to find that many of the plants that we now cultivate purely because they're ornamental were once highly regarded not for their looks but for their flavour. Many of our garden favourites, primped and pushed and preened and trained not to slouch at county shows, are equally at home in dishes in other parts of the world. Hosta, for example, is known as *urui* in Japan and served with sesame sauce; sumac, a lovely ornamental tree seen in many gardens, yields an exotic spice that can be bought in the souks of Istanbul. Pyracantha (firethorn), so common that I'd happily bet you've got one growing within a few metres of your house, yields berries which were once a popular ingredient in both sweet and savoury dishes in the UK. Much of this, I suspect, is down to fashion; food fads come and go.

Where our indigenous wild plants carry with them charming stories and superstitions, and have old wives' tales and folk names attached to them which give a clue as to their uses and form part of our genetic memory, the plants that we think of as 'cultivated', and which the major part of this book deals with, tend to come from other, foreign places and don't have quite the same threads of nostalgia for us. And yet they too have their stories, though they belong to different times and to different peoples. After all, every plant on this planet started life as a wild thing; it's when the plant is unfamiliar that it becomes exotic. Having said that, I have included a small number of plants native to the British Isles that are possibly overlooked or misunderstood, such as the strawberry tree (*Arbutus unedo*).

To garden or to cook?

I hope that this book will be a journey of discovery for people who enjoy their garden and cooking. It may not fundamentally alter the way you work either in your garden or in your kitchen, but I do hope it will make you look at things in a different way, and maybe, in your mind, you'll step into the footsteps of different people in different places. And what you'll learn about the plants included here should enhance both your cooking and your gardening, as well as contribute to your general health and well-being. Nutritionists tell us that we need to eat 30 different foodstuffs per day, and if a small handful of these can come from your garden or window box, then so much the better.

About the plants

I have listed each plant according to its most commonly known name, followed by its scientific genus name. Where a particular species is the best one to eat or cook and is illustrated, then that species name is included. So, for example, all hostas are edible, so the common name (hosta) is followed only by the genus name (*Hosta*). In the case of lavender, the Latin genus name, *Lavandula*, is followed by the species name *angustifolia*, which is one of the nicest kinds to eat. Other edible varieties will be mentioned in the text. Wherever you see the word *edulis* applied to any plant, this means that the plant is edible. In some rare instances, strains of a particular plant are not edible, and this is also made clear in the text.

Unless you are absolutely certain what plant you are dealing with, don't eat it. When trying new plant foods for the first time, follow the same rules as for any new food; only try a little to make sure that you like it and that it agrees with you.

All of the plants included in this book were available at one or other of just two garden centres near my home in Wales, and although passion flower would benefit from the heat of a conservatory, for the most part I have chosen plants that are hardy and easy to grow. However, if you want to buy ornamental plants specifically to eat, unless you can be certain that the grower has organic certification, then you will need to wait two seasons for the plant to be rid of any trace chemical fertilisers or insecticides. Similarly, if you look over the fence and see that your neighbour has a fine crop of something you'd like to try, make sure that the plant has not been treated with any chemicals. It is very likely that you'll have many of the plants mentioned in this book either in your garden or close by

(berberis, rose and pyracantha are three that spring to mind immediately).

Useful equipment and tips

For the most part, the recipes in this book do not require any equipment that's beyond the range of even the most basic kitchen. Several times, however, I specify the use of a non-reactive pan. This means a pan made of a material that will not leave a residual flavour or taint; Pyrex or stainless-steel pans are fine, but aluminium is not.

There are several recipes for jams and jelly where a sugar thermometer would be handy but not essential: if you don't have one you can test for setting point using the old-fashioned 'cold saucer' test. Put a couple of saucers into the freezer, and when your jam has cooked for long enough put a small blob on to the saucer and leave for a few seconds. Push the blob gently with your finger; if it wrinkles, then the jam is ready. Other useful jam- and jelly-making equipment includes a decent wide, heavy-bottomed pan, lidded jam jars and waxed discs, a fine-meshed sieve and a jelly bag and stand. A jam funnel is not necessary but is useful, as is a maslin pan, which has measurements marked on the inside; very handy when you need to calculate juice volume to sugar ratios, as with jellies. None of this equipment need be expensive. (By the way, if you are planning to sell your jams and jellies then you are required by law to use brand-new containers.) If you're making jam for your own consumption, wash jars and their lids carefully in hot, soapy water, rinse, then dry upside down on a lined baking tray in the oven at 170°C/gas 3 for 10 minutes. This sterilises the jars. Always put warm liquid into warm jars, and cold into cold.

For any of the wine recipes, you will need a food-grade plastic container with a lid, demijohns, airlocks and bungs, a funnel and the same straining bag that you use for jam.

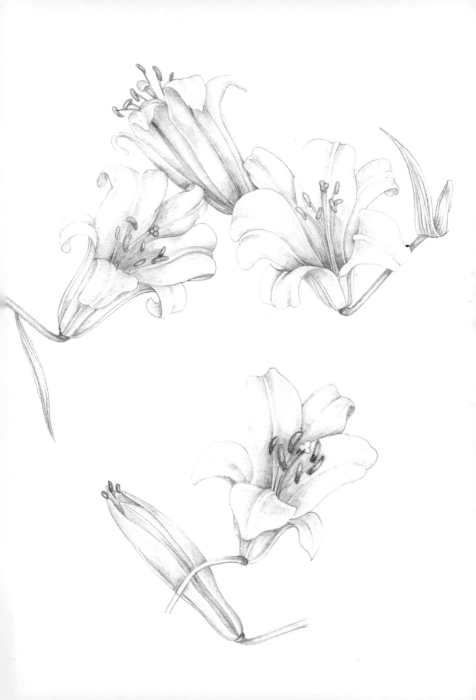

Amaranth

Amaranthus caudatus

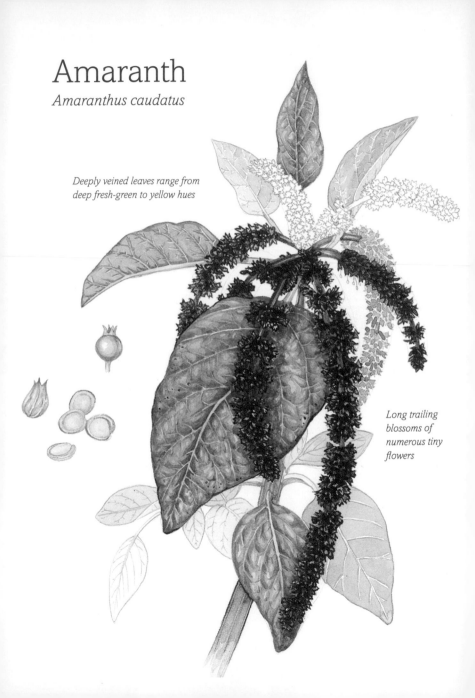

Deeply veined leaves range from deep fresh-green to yellow hues

Long trailing blossoms of numerous tiny flowers

The name amaranth is derived from Greek, and means 'unfading flower'; perhaps that's why it is also a symbol of everlasting life and carries connotations of longevity for various organisations (such as the Order of the Amaranth, a female Masonic society) that bear its name today. The amaranth originates in South America, where the seeds of the plant were such an important dietary staple for the Aztecs that they honoured the tiny grains by mixing them with honey (or blood) and fashioned them into statues of their primary deity, the hummingbird warrior Huitzilopochtli. Just like the Christian act of Communion, in which bread is broken and shared, the statues were cut into pieces so that everyone could consume a little of their god. *A. caudatus* is also known as 'love-lies-bleeding', a lyrical description of the distinctive dangling tassels of blood-red flowers, which will grow to 45cm in length. A half-hardy annual shrub, the amaranth will grow to 1.2m tall in a good, well-drained and fertile soil. In milder areas, love-lies-bleeding will self-seed prolifically, but with such a pretty plant this is no bad thing. It doesn't respond well to being moved, but grows easily from seed. Try planting it together with Joseph's coat (*A. tricolor*), each leaf of which is a carnival of red, green and yellow; hence the

name, in honour of the biblical character's garment.

Common Names and Species

Love-lies-bleeding, tassel flower, pendant amaranth. Other names for different cultivars – of which there are many – include Joseph's coat (*A. tricolor*), pigweed (*A. albus*), Prince of Wales', or, Prince's feather (*A. hypochondriacus*) and Chinese spinach (*A. dubius* or *yin choy*).

Medicinal Use

Amaranth is rich in nutrients and has many health benefits. Native American tribes used the cooked leaves of amaranth as a cure for constipation; modern-day herbalists use it to treat gastroenteritis and diarrhoea. Amaranth seeds contain a compound called 'squalene', which the Native Americans called *samaweda*, meaning 'cure-all'. Squalene has antioxidant properties, which are known to be useful in the battle against cancer.

Culinary Use

Amaranth is typical of a plant that westerners regard as purely ornamental, but if you are in any doubt as to its edibility, then the many names by which it is known around the world are testimony to its tastiness. In India, amaranth greens go by many names, including *chaulai*, *chua*, *cheera*, *keerai* and *harive*; in Malaysia and Indonesia it can be found in the markets under the title of *bayam*; in China it appears on the menu as *yin choy*, or Chinese spinach; and in Vietnam, you can eat *rau den* soup. In Africa, it goes by several different names, too, including *chewa*, *embu* and *meru*, and in Jamaica it goes by the best of all the names, in my opinion, *callaloo*, and is sold in tins. One of the simplest ways of cooking your amaranth leaves is as *vleeta*, a Greek dish where the leaves are wilted then dressed with olive oil and lemon, and served with a heap of sliced fried potatoes on the side.

The flavour of the leaves and stems is like a slightly sweeter version of spinach, and it marries well with spices. If you'd like to try the seeds, the renowned American wild-food expert Euell Gibbons recommends gathering the seeds, spreading them on a plastic sheet and walking across them to crush the shells. Then gather the shiny black seeds and roast them in a slow oven before pounding into a fine, dark meal to add flavour to baking.

I chose this particular amaranth (*A. caudatus*) as an illustration because it is one of the most popular of the species and therefore the one you'll find most easily, although all cultivars can be used in the same way; i.e. all parts of the plant – the seeds, leaves and stems – are edible and not only tasty but very nutritious, too.

Jamaican Calalloo

Serves 4–6 as a side dish

10 sprigs (150–200g) fresh amaranth leaves
1 onion, chopped
1 large ripe tomato, chopped
1 teaspoon finely chopped fresh thyme or ½ teaspoon dried thyme
½ scotch bonnet chilli, deseeded and finely chopped
200ml coconut milk
salt and pepper, to taste
15g butter

Wash the amaranth leaves thoroughly and remove any tough stems, then rip or slice into fine shreds.

Put the leaves in a pan and add the onion, tomato, thyme, chilli and coconut milk. Season well with salt and pepper. Cover and cook over a low heat for about 45 minutes. Taste and add more seasoning if necessary.

Before serving, stir in the butter. Serve with chunks of crusty bread or rice.

Keralan Cheera Thoran

Thoran is a dry vegetable curry from Kerala in south-west India and is usually served as part of a *Sadya*, or celebration feast.

Serves 4 as a main dish, or 6–8 as a side dish

3 large handfuls of amaranth (cheera) leaves
salt, to taste
a generous glug of vegetable oil
½ teaspoon yellow mustard seeds
250g shallot, thinly sliced
5 garlic cloves, crushed or finely chopped
a sprig of fresh or dried curry leaves
4 dried chillies, roughly chopped
150ml water

For the curry paste
250g freshly grated coconut
2 fresh green chillies, finely chopped
a pinch of turmeric
¼ teaspoon cumin powder

First make the curry paste. Grind the coconut, chillies, turmeric and cumin into a rough paste with a pestle and mortar or in a blender. Set aside.

Wash the amaranth leaves and remove any tough stalks, then chop them roughly. Put the leaves in a bowl and stir in a little salt to taste.

Heat the oil in a heavy-bottomed frying pan (with a lid). Add the mustard seeds and when they're sputtering, add the shallot, garlic, curry leaves and chillies. Turn down the heat slightly and fry for a few minutes, stirring. Add the amaranth leaves, water and a sprinkle of salt and cook for 5 minutes, stirring so that it doesn't catch and burn. When the water has nearly all evaporated, add the curry paste and stir to mix well. Cover the pan, then turn the heat down to very low and cook for a further 5 minutes. Taste to ensure that the leaves are cooked. Remove the lid and, if necessary, cook down further until the mixture is dry.

Serve with rice and *roti*.

Astilbe

Astilbe thunbergii

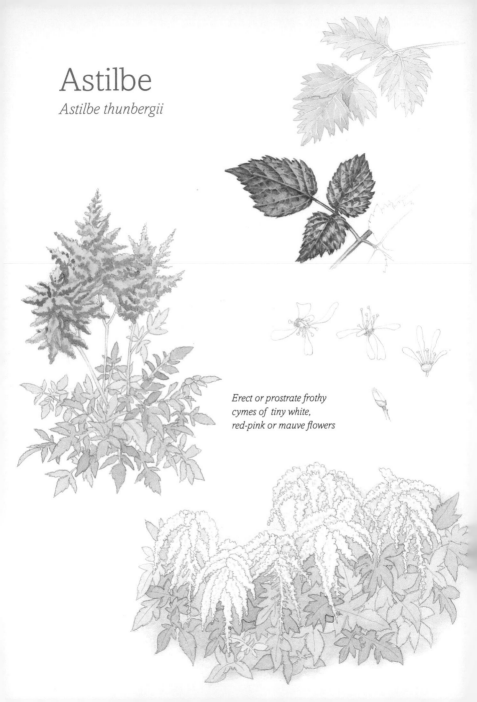

*Erect or prostrate frothy
cymes of tiny white,
red-pink or mauve flowers*

Astilbe is from the Greek *'a'*, meaning 'without', and *stilbe*, 'brilliance', thus 'without brilliance'. This refers to each tiny little flower – only 3mm or so in diameter – which is quite insignificant. However, as a mass, they're really quite impressive.

This particular plant, very common in gardens, originated in North America and in East Asia/China. Astilbe looks very similar to the wild meadowsweet (*Filipendula ulmaria*). Meadowsweet, confusingly, is also one of the nicknames for astilbe. The two plants are actually distantly related. Astilbe blossoms in the summer with frothy panicles of thousands of tiny flowers contributing to a pretty, delicate candy-floss-like texture, often shaped as a distinctive plumy, feathery spire. The flowers come in a whole spectrum of colours from a creamy white through to pinks, reds and purples. Although there are as yet no cultivars bearing yellow flowers, the leaves range from the darkest green to the palest lime/yellow. Astilbes are hardy herbaceous perennials, meaning that they will stay put and flower for you year after year so long as conditions are right. The plants like moist, rich, peaty soil and partial shade, although in my experience they don't seem to mind their roots being slightly fried in hot, dry weather. They don't like lime. Although some varieties are small,

growing to a height of only 15cm, some can grow up to 1.5m tall, so the plumes of flowers are immediately recognisable from a distance and form a perfect foil to the more sculptural plants in a flower border. Left in the ground to dry out, the plants will give you a beautiful winter display, too; frost-touched ghosts on a winter morning.

Common Names
False goat's beard, false spirea and (sometimes) meadowsweet.

Medicinal Use
During the Tang dynasty (the eighth century) the dried roots of the *A. thunbergii* variety were used to heal open wounds, even those caused by sword injuries. Interestingly, recent studies suggest that the plant does indeed have compounds that can help to heal wounds. Today, we have the technology to be able to determine such uses of plants, but information like this wasn't available back then.

Culinary Use
Not all parts of the astilbe are edible, but you might like to try the tender young shoots of the *A. thunbergii* species. The shoots have a delicate, celery-like flavour and can be simply steamed with a little butter, salt and pepper to allow you to appreciate the

flavour of what, for most people, will be an unusual ingredient. The older leaves, dried, make an acceptable alternative to black tea, although it's the *A. longicarpa* species that is traditionally used for this purpose. Simply pick the leaves on a dry, sunny day and dry them in a dehydrator or put them in a paper bag and hang in a warm, dry place until crisp. Use half a teaspoonful per cup or to taste.

Astilbe Iced Tea

A perfect drink for a summer's day.

Serves 8

4 teaspoons dried astilbe leaves
1 litre boiling water
4 tablespoons soft brown sugar
a handful of mint leaves, torn
crushed ice
juice of 2 large oranges
juice of 1 lemon
mint sprigs and lemon slices, to garnish

Put the dried, crumbled leaves into a heatproof jug and pour the boiling water over them. Leave for 5 minutes, then strain the tea into a separate jug and discard the leaves. Add the soft brown sugar, then stir until the sugar has dissolved and leave to cool.

Mix together the torn mint and the ice. Half-fill tall glasses with the ice, orange and lemon juice and mint and top up with the tea. Garnish each glass with a sprig of mint and a slice of lemon.

Tea Loaf with Astilbe

Makes 6–8 slices

350g mixed dried fruit
2 tablespoons freshly brewed tea made
*   with 2 teaspoons dried astilbe leaves*
*   (see recipe opposite)*
2 medium eggs, beaten
200g soft light-brown sugar
270g self-raising flour
2 teaspoons ground cinnamon or
*   mixed spice*

Put the fruit into a bowl and add the hot astilbe-leaf tea. Leave overnight, by which time the fruit will have soaked up all the liquid.

Preheat the oven to 170°C/gas 3. Line a 23cm loaf tin with baking parchment or greaseproof paper.

Add the eggs to the soaked fruit. Stir in the sugar, sift in the flour and the spice and mix well with a wooden spoon (or use an electric mixer). Spoon into the lined loaf tin and bake, turning the tin halfway through the cooking time so that the loaf bakes evenly, for 60–75 minutes or until an inserted skewer comes out clean.

Leave to cool completely before removing from the cake tin.

This is a moist loaf cake that will not need butter. Wrapped in foil and stored in an airtight tin, it should keep for up to 2 weeks.

Autumn Olive

Elaeagnus umbellata

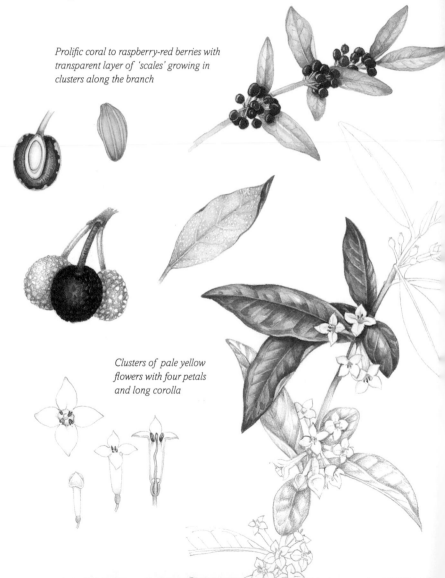

Prolific coral to raspberry-red berries with transparent layer of 'scales' growing in clusters along the branch

Clusters of pale yellow flowers with four petals and long corolla

The name *elaeagnus* actually means 'sacred olive' (from the Greek *elaia*, meaning 'olive tree', and *agnos*, meaning 'sacred'). In Iranian and Persian cooking, the fruit of this small tree or shrub is known as senjed, or wild lotus fruit; if you have access to a Middle Eastern grocery or deli, or if you happen to be in Iran, you will find packets of senjed berries for sale. Legend has it that if you fall asleep under the senjed tree, then you will become oblivious of anything but the dream world. The tree itself symbolises both passion and beauty, and the fruits (dried and ground to a powder) are often used as one of the seven ingredients of Norooz, the Persian New Year, celebrating the start of a brand-new year filled with fun, food, family and music.

Most of the *Elaeagnus* species we see today originated in Asia; however, the plant has had no problem in adapting to conditions all over Europe, the UK, US and even Australia. The berries belonging to the *E. multiflora* and *E. umbellata* (illustrated opposite) species are by far the tastiest and juiciest and where the plant is cultivated for the fruit, these are the most common choices; others, such as those of *E. angustifolia*, tend to be on the dry side – but are still good for making into jams, jellies and wines. And when the berries appear, they are abundant. The most common

species in the US is *E. commutata*, the American silverberry or wolf willow.

Despite its exotic origins, elaeagnus is one of those serviceable but often overlooked shrubs, frequently used in municipal planting, hedging and the like. Elaeagnus can be evergreen or deciduous, appearing either as a shrub or as a small tree. One of its folk names is silverthorn, which refers to the teeny silver-brown scales that cover the shoots and undersides of the leaves. The 'thorn' part of the name is a bit misleading, since the plant doesn't have thorns so much as sharpish young twigs that later develop into branches. The flowers are tiny and white, and although their appearance might be insignificant, the fragrance is another matter; blooming in autumn, the flowers are highly aromatic and their honey-like scent fills the garden at this time. Wherever elaeagnus is deliberately planted, this is mainly for its attractive, dense, shiny, sometimes variegated leaves.

Elaeagnus is so adaptable that in some cases the plant is regarded as invasive (indeed, in Massachusetts and New Hampshire it's listed as a prohibited plant). It will withstand harsh weather, including salt-laden sea winds, cold conditions (although not arctic) and poor soils. It will withstand drought, too, but being waterlogged is a definite no-no. One of the classic plants used in perma-culture, elaeagnus has no problem with being cut or pruned, hence its suitability as boundary hedging. It also takes well to bonsai treatment. An added bonus for gardeners considering whether or not to add an elaeagnus to their plot is that it fixes nitrogen into the soil, meaning that poor soil poses no problems for the plant. Often, the plant is spread by its seeds after they have been eaten (and subsequently distributed in the traditional manner) by birds.

Common Names and Species
Silverthorn (*E. pungens*), thorny olive, thorny silverberry, spreading oleaster, Russian olive, American silverberry, wolf willow (*E. commutata*), *E. angustifolia*, *E. multiflora*.

Medicinal Use
Elaeagnus fruits are rich in vitamin C and are used to treat coughs, colds and flu. Unusually for a fruit, elaeagnus also contains essential fatty acids. It is currently being investigated for its potential to reduce incidences of cancer as well as the possibility of halting or reversing the growth of cancer cells.

Culinary Use
Unripe elaeagnus fruit is generally a bit on the tart side for most taste buds. The ripe berries, however, are deliciously sharp and sweet plucked straight from the bush, with a flavour somewhere between a cherry and a tart grape. When they're ripe, the berries should simply drop into your hand from the branch. Inside the fruit is a kernel, which is also edible.

Native American tribes in Alaska used to eat the entire fruit, including the little nut, fried in moose fat. You could also dry the berries after removing the kernel, either in a dehydrator or in a very low oven, then store them in jars and use in muffins or fruit cakes. You might also like to make a delicious 'cherry' brandy.

Autumn-Olive Brandy

Makes 75cl

Decant half a litre of brandy into a clean 1 litre bottle, add enough elaeagnus fruit to fill the bottle to three-quarters full, then add golden caster sugar almost to the top, leaving a 3cm or so gap, so that you can shake the contents of the bottle. Leave to infuse in a cool, dark place for 6 months. Strain the brandy into a fresh, clean bottle.

Spicy Autumn-Olive Ketchup

Makes 500ml

500g elaeagnus fruit
300ml water
170g dark muscovado sugar
300ml cider vinegar
3cm fresh root ginger, grated
1 fresh red chilli
½ teaspoon salt
½ teaspoon freshly ground pepper

Wash the fruit and put in a large pan with the water. Simmer for about 20 minutes, or until the fruits easily come away from the seeds. Leave to cool slightly, then press through a fine-meshed sieve to remove the seeds and tougher bits of skin.

Put the fruit pulp in a pan over a medium heat and cook, stirring constantly, for about 5 minutes, until the colour darkens.

Add the sugar, vinegar, ginger and chilli and heat gently until the sugar has dissolved. Take off the heat, remove the chilli if you wish, then use a stick blender to blend to a very smooth paste. Return to the heat and bring to the boil, stirring, and cook for 5 minutes to reduce to the gloopy consistency of ketchup. Season well.

Leave to cool, then pour into sterilised jars or bottles and seal. The ketchup will keep, refrigerated, for up to 6 months.

Bamboo

Phyllostachys edulis

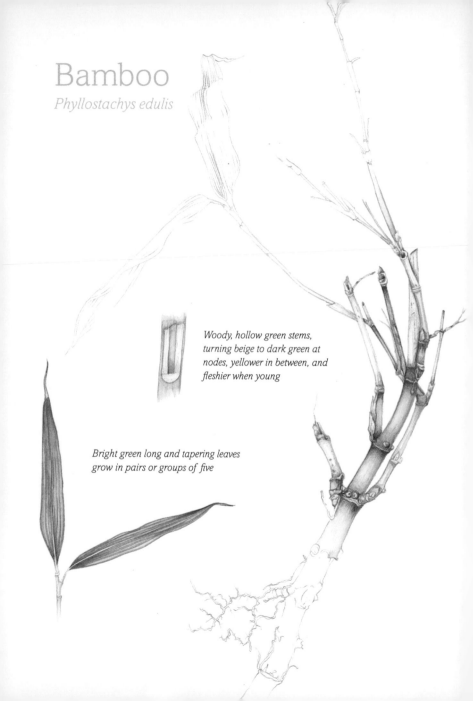

Woody, hollow green stems,
turning beige to dark green at
nodes, yellower in between, and
fleshier when young

Bright green long and tapering leaves
grow in pairs or groups of five

Bamboo belongs to the same family as grass and, despite the disparity in size, you can see the similarities; both are tall, fast-growing, jointed plants of vigorous habit. Indigenous to East Asia, India, Africa and parts of southern America, bamboo might not be native to Europe, but it certainly grows well in cooler climates. If you have never had bamboo in your garden and fancy some, think carefully about where you will plant it: it can become very invasive and hard to get rid of.

Bamboo is one of the many plants on this earth that has had a major role in the lives of human beings; its uses are phenomenally varied. In India, Japan and China bows and arrows were made of bamboo, as were sharp-tipped spears. And prior to paper, bamboo was used as a writing material by the Chinese. For thousands of years, bamboo has been used to make containers, cooking implements, furniture, boats and even bridges and buildings. In fact, wherever you live there's likely to be something in your home made from bamboo (I'm looking at a bamboo chair here in Wales), and who hasn't had bamboo roller blinds at some time in their life? Bamboo fabric, which is becoming more widely available these days, is satisfyingly heavy and unexpectedly silky-soft to the touch.

Bamboo has symbolic meanings, too, largely related to its prodigious growth and its tenacity. The bamboo groves around Shinto shrines are there to protect the holy place from evil spirits, which are said to become entangled in the tall, dense thickets. That the roots of individual stems of bamboo become entwined, making them strong enough to help some buildings withstand earthquakes, further underlines the symbolism of the plant as a protective force. However, while some western exponents of feng shui might grow bamboo close to their houses for this reason, they find that the roots can sometimes undermine the foundations of brick houses; superstitions may be charming but not when they supersede common sense. Houses in Europe are, after all, on the whole less prone to earthquakes than those in Asia.

Common Names and Species
Sweetshoot bamboo (*P. dulcis*).

Medicinal Use
As a medicinal plant, bamboo is surprisingly useful too. Among other things, it is rich in calcium, iron and vitamin C; at one time, bamboo roots were used as a cure for rabies but there is no clinical evidence to support this treatment. Another folk use of bamboo leaves was as an aphrodisiac – again, there is no proof of its

effectiveness, but you could always give it a go. Throughout parts of Asia the young shoots are infused in water and used as a gargle to combat respiratory problems such as asthma.

Culinary Use

The good news is that if you do happen to have a surfeit of bamboo in your garden, then eating it is as good a way as any to arrest its progress. The other good news is that all types of bamboo are edible; some, however, are tastier than others and some also need to be boiled to remove any possible irritants. It's the young shoots that you're after. Among the species that are very good indeed to eat are *P. edulis* (*edulis* means 'edible') and *P. dulcis* (*dulcis* means 'sweet'). The popularity of the shoots as a foodstuff is reflected in its many different names (*rebung* in Malaysia and India, *mama* in Vietnam and *tama* in Nepal are just a few of many) and also in the number of dishes that use them.

How to Prepare Bamboo Shoots

The young shoots need to be picked before they reach 30cm in height. Slice them from the base of the plant, using a very sharp knife; you will be astonished at how tough the stems are. Although the shoots of the plants mentioned above are so sweet that they can be eaten raw, others need to be cooked to remove bitterness before using. It's the tender creamy white inner part of the stem that is used. If they are very bitter, cut them into slices, then cover with water and leave in the fridge for three days until the bitterness has leached away. Alternatively, after gathering, slice off the ends, any tough outer leaves and the sheath. Add to a pan of boiling water and boil for up to 25 minutes – the bigger the shoot, the longer you'll need to cook it to remove the bitter taste – then slice into regular, oblong strips.

Sour and Spicy Noodle Soup with Bamboo Shoots

Serves 4

For the soup
1 tablespoon vegetable oil
3cm fresh root ginger, thinly sliced
250g fresh shitake mushrooms,
   thinly sliced
1 fresh red chilli, finely chopped
1 tablespoon dark soy sauce
1 tablespoon light soy sauce
1 tablespoon balsamic vinegar
1 tablespoon Chinese rice wine
700ml vegetable stock
220g bamboo shoots, cooked
   as described opposite and
   thinly sliced
pepper, to taste
1 tablespoon cornflour, mixed
   to a paste with 2 tablespoons
   cold water

For the noodles
200g egg noodles, cooked
200g fresh beansprouts
2 spring onions, sliced on the diagonal

To make the soup, heat the oil in a large, heavy-bottomed pan or wok, then fry the ginger and the mushrooms for a couple of minutes until soft. Add the chilli, dark and light soy sauce, balsamic vinegar, rice wine, stock and the cooked bamboo shoots, season with pepper and bring to the boil. Lower the heat and simmer for 10 minutes to allow the flavours to deepen. Remove from the heat and stir in the cornflour paste. Return to the heat, and cook, stirring until the broth has thickened slightly.

Divide the cooked noodles between four bowls, pour the broth over the noodles and sprinkle a handful of beansprouts and spring-onion slices over each portion.

Serves 4

1 tablespoon vegetable oil
150g onions, chopped
3cm fresh root ginger, grated
1 medium fresh red chilli, chopped
1 teaspoon cumin powder
½ teaspoon turmeric
250g black-eyed beans, soaked
*   overnight*
300g potatoes, cooked and cut
*   into 2cm cubes*
250g bamboo shoots
150g ripe tomatoes, chopped
salt and pepper, to taste
a handful of coriander, chopped

Heat the oil in a frying pan and sauté the onions until golden, before adding all the spices. Stir for a couple of minutes to release the flavours, then add the black-eyed beans, the potatoes and the bamboo shoots. Stir for 2–3 minutes before adding the chopped tomatoes and a little water if necessary. Season well. Cover and cook until the beans are tender. Just before serving, stir in the coriander. Serve with rice.

Bee Balm

Monarda didyma

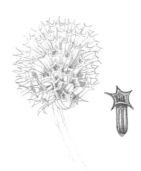

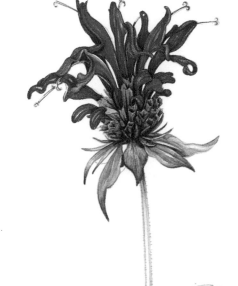

Flowers range from orange, scarlet, pale pink to magenta with sepals of similar shade to flower

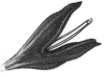

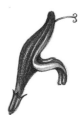

Paired, opposite, oblong leaves with toothed margins

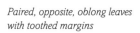

A member of the mint family, bee balm is often overlooked and yet it's a very pretty garden flower which has the added benefit of being edible. And bees love it. Bee balm is native to North America. The Oswego tribes of Native Americans made a tea from the leaves of the plant and this flavoursome drink was quickly adopted by the European settlers. However, bee balm mustn't be confused with the bergamot orange, which is used to flavour Earl Grey tea. The two plants are not related, although the similarity of the scent gives rise to the wild-bergamot epithet.

Bee balm is a hardy, clump-forming perennial, which can grow to 1.5m in height, given the right conditions. These include moist soil and either full sunshine or partial shade; edges of woodlands suit the plant as well as the formal flower bed. In bloom in summer, its unusual, tufty flowers with tubular petals give them something of the appearance of a butterfly. The flowers of bee balm come in a whole spectrum of colours from a creamy white through to pinks, reds and dark purples. The leaves are long and narrow with small serrated edges not unlike those of nettles or mint.

Common Names
Wild bergamot, crimson or scarlet bee balm, horsemint, oswego (or Oswego tea), golden melissa, Indian nettle.

Medicinal Use
Native Americans used bee balm to fight an array of different ailments and it was they who introduced this aspect of the herb to the settlers. Bee balm can aid digestion and bring down a fever. It is also strongly antiseptic and contains thymol, an ingredient that appears in commercial mouthwashes and toothpastes. Butterflies and bees love the flower and if you happen to get stung, a poultice of the bee-balm leaves and flowers will soothe the pain – hence the name.

Culinary Use
The leaves, petals and stems of bee balm have a minty scent and flavour with a warming, spicy tang. The flavour of the flowers is more delicate than that of the leaves. You can add the shredded petals and leaves to salads – but bear in mind that a little goes a long way. Similarly, mix them into plain yoghurt and add some freshly squeezed orange juice, for an interesting salsa to go with grilled fish. The flowers are lovely stirred into cream cheese, then piled on to rye bread and topped with slices of cucumber, for a summery snack. You can also flavour a plain sponge cake or muffins by stirring a scattering of the fresh petals into the dough.

Bee-Balm, Coconut and Cashew Chutney

Serves 4

100g fresh young bee-balm leaves
  and flower petals
2 tablespoons cashew nuts, plus
  a few to garnish
1 fresh red chilli
1cm fresh root ginger, grated
a pinch of cumin
50g coconut cream
a large pinch of sea salt and pepper
1 teaspoon soft brown sugar
juice of 2 lemons
50g shredded coconut

Pick over and wash the leaves and petals.

Dry-roast the nuts in a heavy-bottomed pan, shaking the pan continuously so they don't burn. Allow to cool.

Put the roasted nuts, chilli, ginger and cumin into a blender and whizz for a few seconds before adding the coconut cream, salt, pepper and sugar. Add a little water (not too much – you can always add a little more but you can't take any away). Blend thoroughly, stopping to scrape the mixture from the sides of the blender if necessary. Add the bee-balm leaves and lemon juice and whizz again. Scoop into a bowl and stir in the coconut shreds and bee-balm petals, distributing them evenly. Serve immediately.

This is delicious with noodles and a little sesame oil or with crackers and a mild cream cheese.

Begonia

Begonia

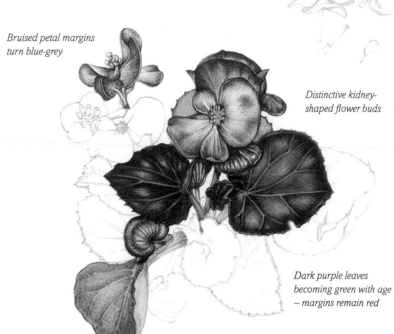

Bruised petal margins
turn blue-grey

Distinctive kidney-
shaped flower buds

Dark purple leaves
becoming green with age
– margins remain red

Anthers swollen and
golden, becoming thin
and orange with age

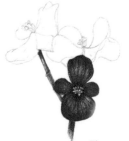

Flower stem matches
flower colour

The Grateful Dead are, as far as I can ascertain, the only rockers to feature the name of this flower in a song title. 'Scarlet Begonias' contains some immortal lines (which I can only paraphrase here for fear of being taken to court) about a girl, like no other girl, who not only likes to wear rings on her fingers and bells on her toes, but caps the whole hippy ensemble by wearing scarlet begonias in her hair ...

For those of you who subscribe to the ancient Persian wisdom that flowers carry meanings (a concept eagerly embraced by enthusiastic and imaginative Victorian ladies and gents) you'll be grateful to know that if you receive a gift of begonias, then the bearer may be trying to tell you, 'BEWARE! I am fanciful!' Then again, it's probably that he or she may have no idea of this obscure little warning.

Begonias proliferate naturally in damp, subtropical climates, including Africa, South and Central America and parts of Asia, including North Korea where the begonia is the national flower. The first European to 'discover' the *Begonia* genus was a French monk, Charles Plumier, something of a polymath, who later became Royal Botanist to King Louis XIV. It was during a trip in 1689–90 to the French Antilles, including Haiti, that Plumier made one of the 1,400 or so plant discoveries of his illustrious career; he diplomatically named the begonia after the then-governor of Haiti, Michel Begon.

Medicinal Use

A good source of vitamin C, all parts of begonias used to be eaten to combat scurvy. In the West Indies, herbalists use begonia roots to treat cancer, although this has not been subjected to conclusive testing. In China, at one time, the flower had medicinal as well as edible uses; it was made into medicines that had a variety of applications, including disinfecting wounds, curing kidney ailments, soothing burns, preventing colds and even fixing toothache.

Culinary Use

The group of plants covered by the name begonia is many and varied: evergreen or deciduous, cane-stemmed, summer flowering or winter flowering, perennial or annual. The last are the ones that most of us are acquainted with, to be seen proliferating in window boxes and flower beds. These are in the group known as tuberous begonias, often bought as showy bedding plants. They have quite large flowers looking not dissimilar to unfurled roses. The stems, leaves and petals of the begonia can be eaten. You can nibble on the petals as an addition to a salad or, if you really wanted to, you could even make cheese, using the sap of the tuberous begonia to curdle the milk. The leaves and petals have a refreshing, sharply acidic flavour, and the stems can be used exactly like rhubarb and make a great, tart addition to a smoothie; try strawberry, banana, mango, plain yoghurt and a few begonia stems to add bite and piquancy. You can also fry the leaves just as you would chips. The leaves will turn black, but don't worry; serve with salt and pepper.

Begonia, Strawberry and Peach Crumble

Serves 4

For the crumble topping
140g flour (plain or self-raising)
100g golden caster sugar
50g desiccated coconut
100g butter, chilled and diced,
  plus extra for greasing
100g pomegranate seeds,
  for sprinkling

For the fruit
300g begonia stems, chopped into
  3cm lengths
100g golden caster sugar, plus 50g
  for topping the crumble mix
¼ teaspoon vanilla extract
300g ripe strawberries, halved
300g ripe peaches, peeled, stoned
  and quartered

Preheat the oven to 190°C/gas 5. Grease a baking tray and line with parchment paper.

For the topping, tip the flour, sugar and coconut into a bowl and rub in the butter until the mixture resembles fresh breadcrumbs. Tip the mixture on to the prepared baking tray and spread it evenly, then bake in the oven for 10 minutes.

To prepare the fruit, put the begonia stems with 100g sugar, a splash of water and the vanilla extract into a pan. Stir over a gentle heat for 5 minutes, then add the strawberries and peaches and cook for a further 2 minutes (unlike a crumble that uses harder fruit such as apples, you don't want to cook away the texture of the strawberries and peaches).

Put the fruit mixture in an oven-proof dish, top with the crumble, sprinkle the remaining sugar over the top and bake for 15 minutes. Remove from the oven, leave to cool for 10 minutes and then scatter the pomegranate seeds over the top.

Serve with cream, ice-cream or, best of all, elderflower sorbet.

Begonia Vinaigrette

Makes 550ml

1 cup begonia flower petals,
  picked over and washed
1 cup apple juice
1 tablespoon runny honey
1 tablespoon red wine vinegar

Use equal amounts – in volume – of the flowers and the apple juice. This recipe uses a standard mugful (about 250ml) for measuring. Then add a tablespoon each of the runny honey and the vinegar, and blend in a food processor until smooth. Taste, and add more vinegar if you want to use as a thinner salad dressing. This will keep in a clean jar in the fridge; shake before use. It's worth making with the fresh flowers and will store well if refrigerated.

To serve, pour into the 'bowl' of a ripe avocado and add a couple of fresh begonia blossoms and some crisp salad leaves.

Begonia Sandwich or Cake Filling

Makes 375g

225g soft cream cheese
75g strawberry jam or jelly
75g begonia petals and stems,
*   washed and chopped*

Simply stir the cheese and strawberry jam or jelly together thoroughly, then add the chopped begonia. This is delicious in a sandwich made with fresh sourdough bread and works wonderfully as a filling for sponge cake, too.

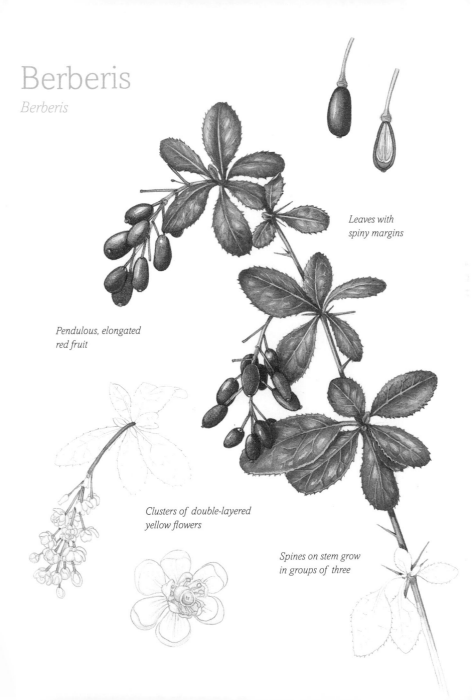

Berberis
Berberis

Leaves with
spiny margins

Pendulous, elongated
red fruit

Clusters of double-layered
yellow flowers

Spines on stem grow
in groups of three

There are over 500 species of berberis growing in every country on the planet, in all climates, apart from Antarctica and Australia. All varieties of berberis are edible. The Oregon grape, also known as mahonia (see page 167), is also a member of the *Berberis* family. Italians call the shrub the holy thorn, since they believe this is the plant that was used to make Christ's crown of thorns. Some varieties, for example *Berberis darwinii*, are indeed hellishly prickly and require thick gauntlets should you need to prune it. While you're pruning, you might notice that the inner part of the woody stems is a bright orange colour. A similarly coloured dye can be made from the plant.

Berberis shrubs come in many varieties. Some sprawl along the ground or up walls and others form densely constructed thickets, hence their popularity as a hedging plant. They're tough and frost-hardy, happy to grow in all sorts of soil and weather conditions, propagating themselves very effectively (rather too effectively, according to some) by throwing out suckers. Berberis flowers appear either singly or in dangling racemes of yellow or orange blossoms, and the ripe berries vary in colour from red to dark purple and can be either rounded or distinctly oval-shaped.

Common Names and Species

Barberry, *zereshk*, pipperidges, holy thorn, *Berberis vulgaris* (see illustration on page 41).

Medicinal Use

The compound berberine, extracted from the *B. vulgaris* species, is effective in treating polycystic ovary syndrome.

Culinary Use

Of late, the little berries of this bush – called barberries – have become something of an exotic food trend. If you're browsing in a deli – or, more likely, in an Iranian grocery – you might come across packs of them. The Iranians call them *zereshk*. They don't come cheap in their dried form and if you manage to find them fresh then they're even more expensive.

Chances are, though, that you'll be able to access your own fresh *zereshk* much more easily (and economically) closer to home. For example, in the short lane that runs from the back of a friend's house to the main road I recently counted four different shrubs and I bet that none of the owners realise just what a gem they have. All berberis berries are edible, but the most commonly used ones tend to be those of the *B. vulgaris* species (although *B. darwinii* comes close in the popularity stakes for gardeners).

Dorothy Hartley, in her 1953 book

Food in England, writes about them in such a casual way that suggests they must have been so common as to need no explanation. As far back as Elizabethan times they went by the delightfully quaint name of pipperages. But, for some reason, we seem to have neglected them in Britain in recent years. Not so, though, in Russia, where children enjoy a barberry candy, or in Argentina, Chile or Patagonia where the berries are made into jams or jellies; indeed, the plant is the national symbol of Patagonia where, they say, eating just one berry guarantees you a return trip to the country.

Barberries have a delicious citrusy tang; it's worth building up a store of these useful fruits and they are very easy to preserve.

Drying Barberries

Remove any woody bits of twig from the berries. Wash and dry the berries, then spread over newspaper and leave in a warm, dry place for a couple of days until the skins have started to wrinkle. If they happen to be a species that has seeds (check them), slice the side of the berry with a small, very sharp knife and scrape out the seeds (if you leave a few it doesn't matter), then leave to dry again. When they are thoroughly dried, store either in an airtight jar or freeze in airtight bags. You can now use them as 'currants' in sweet dishes or in cakes, and also in savoury meals; traditionally, dried barberries, rehydrated by soaking in water for a few hours, are used with saffron to flavour rice. They can also be ground up with sea salt as a rub for lamb or poultry or used, either rehydrated or fresh, along with pomegranate seeds, to jewel pilaffs.

French Barberry Marmalade
(Marmelade d'épine-vinette)

An old recipe from Rouen for an unusual, rich, dark and delicious marmalade.

Makes 2 x 450g jars

2kg fresh barberries
750g white granulated sugar per 1kg
    cooked barberry pulp (see method)
juice of 1 lemon

Wash the berries and remove the leaves, stalks and twigs. Put the fruit in a heavy-bottomed pan (with a lid), just cover with water and bring to a slow simmer. Cover and simmer for 30 minutes until the fruits can be squished easily with a spoon. Drain the fruit, reserving the liquid, then push the stewed fruit through a fine-meshed sieve to remove any pips. Use a metal spoon to press the fruit through the sieve, scraping the spoon across the underneath of the sieve from time to time to remove the pulp. Stir the reserved stewing liquid back into the pulp and weigh. Weigh the sugar as instructed above.

If you have one, clip a sugar thermometer to the inside of the pan. Put the fruit pulp, sugar and lemon juice into the pan and bring to the boil, stirring constantly so that the mixture doesn't catch. Turn up the heat and cook for about 20 minutes until the mixture reaches 105°C, or setting point. If you don't have a sugar thermometer, use the cold saucer test (see page 13).

Leave to cool slightly, then pour into warm, sterilised jars.

Zereshk Rice Pilaff

Serves 4–6

225g basmati rice
1–2 tablespoons vegetable oil
1 onion, finely chopped
1 garlic clove, crushed
1 large carrot, grated
1 teaspoon cumin seeds
2 teaspoons ground coriander
2 teaspoons black mustard seeds
450ml vegetable stock
4 cardamom pods
75g zereshk
75g unsalted cashew nuts
50g sliced almonds

To garnish
50g pomegranate seeds
chopped fresh coriander

Rinse the rice and drain. Heat the oil in a heavy-bottomed frying pan (with a lid) and sweat the onion, garlic and carrot for 3–4 minutes. Add the spices (except for the cardamom pods) and the rice and stir well to coat the grains with oil. Add the stock and season, then put the cardamom pods on top of the rice (so they will be easy to remove later), bring to the boil and reduce the heat. Cover and simmer gently for 10 minutes. Add the *zereshk* and cook for 5 minutes. Remove from the heat and leave to stand, lid on, for a further 5 minutes.

In the meantime, in a separate, heavy-bottomed pan, dry-toast the nuts lightly, shaking the pan so they don't scorch. This will take only a minute or so.

When the rice has had its standing time, remove the lid, stir and, just before serving, scatter with the toasted nuts, the pomegranate seeds and some fresh coriander.

Birch

Betula

Small, roundish, toothed, pale green leaves ripen to a darker colour by summertime and fade to yellow in autumn

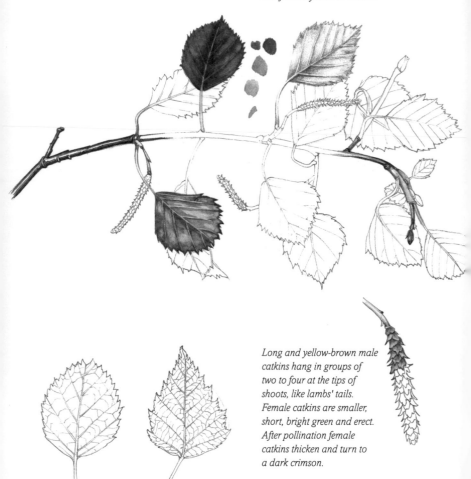

Long and yellow-brown male catkins hang in groups of two to four at the tips of shoots, like lambs' tails. Female catkins are smaller, short, bright green and erect. After pollination female catkins thicken and turn to a dark crimson.

Whether you're a cultivated forager or you prefer the wild stuff, the birch tree is one of the most useful plants you'll find and because these attractive trees often appear in gardens, they merit a place here. There are many different species of birch, which are at home wherever there's a temperate climate. My own particular favourite is the silver birch (*Betula pendula*, otherwise the European birch). Although birches grow so prolifically that some people regard them as weeds, the silver bark with its horizontal black tiger stripes, and the tree's delicate, trailing branches, make the birch exquisitely beautiful. Also, its robust nature as a 'pioneer' tree (able to grow quickly and in poor soil, providing shelter for less hardy trees and plants that need it) makes them even more loveable.

In general, birch trees can grow to about 20m tall and can live for up to 140 years. They like well-drained, slightly acidic soils, and are also quick to colonise scorched or burned ground. They are deciduous, with oval, slightly serrated leaves that begin a pale green in the early spring and ripen to a darker colour by summertime. The word 'birch' comes from a Germanic word meaning 'to shine'; putting the silver birch to one side as an explanation for this descriptive name, I wonder if this might refer also to the leaves, which are very glossy? The trunks of birch trees are striped with distinctive, darker, horizontal lines and the bark itself (specifically, that of the aptly-named paper bark birch) is a very useful material and was even used in centuries past as a form of paper or for making containers, a skill which keen bush crafters keep alive today.

If you suffer from hay fever, it's a pretty good bet that you'd be able to point towards the birch tree as the culprit. Twenty five per cent of sufferers can blame an allergy to birch pollen for this annoying seasonal affliction. Homeopaths believe that a little of the thing that caused the problem can also solve the problem, so it stands to reason that a little birch pollen might alleviate your sneezes. Take a spoonful of honey, dissolve it in a half a cup of warm water. Then take the cup to the birch tree and tap the flower against the inside of the cup, to release a small cloud of pollen. I've been advised that this will work, but as I don't get hay fever I haven't needed to try it for myself.

You can make an interesting birch liqueur by steeping fresh young beech leaves in gin and sugar. Or you can use the leaves and twigs of birch to make a tea – just take six fresh leaves and a 3cm twig to one mug of boiling water, steep for 5 minutes and sweeten to taste. The inner part of the bark can also be eaten raw or can be dried and ground to make flour, which can be added to bulk out normal flour. But by far the tastiest part of the beech tree is its sap, so no apologies for the seeming complexity of the recipe below. This may be a process you enjoy so much that it will become a spring ritual. Any birch tree can be tapped for its sap, but make sure that you cause minimal harm to the tree itself.

Collecting Birch Sap

The window for collecting the birch sap by tapping is quite narrow – about two to three weeks at best – in late winter or early spring, depending on where you live. The sap starts to rise as the days start to get warmer and the average temperature is around 12°C. The larger the crown of the tree, the more sap will be yielded, so avoid younger, smaller trees and don't try to tap a tree with a trunk less than 25cm in diameter. The generally accepted rule is never to tap the same tree two years in a row, nor should you take more than a couple of litres per year from any one tree.

Using a mechanical bit, drill a hole of a scant 3cm deep and no more than 12mm in diameter, angled upwards, at least 1m from the ground. Use a length of food-grade plastic tubing, long enough to reach a clean container placed at ground level; a 2-litre water bottle will do nicely. One end of the tube goes into the hole in the tree, the other goes into the container. Stuff the space around the tube, where the bottle lid should be, with cotton wool or a clean plastic bag. Prop the bottle in such a way that it won't fall over, tying it to the tree if necessary.

The sap will start to drip out within a few minutes, but it's a trickier matter to estimate how long it will take to fill the container – anywhere between 12 and 48 hours, but of course you can collect the sap at any time. When the bottle has filled with sap, remove the tube from the tree, allow any sap that remains in the tube to run into the bottle, then plug the gap in the tree using a new, sterile wine cork cut to fit the hole.

You can drink the sap just as it is, as a spring tonic. The sap is much lighter and thinner than maple syrup but you can reduce it if you prefer a thicker syrup to use on pancakes. The sap is sugar-rich and will want to start fermenting straight away, so you might like to simply go with the flow and make a delicious birch-sap wine. If it's not possible to process the sap as soon as you have harvested it, it will keep, refrigerated, for up to 2 days.

Birch-Sap Wine

Makes enough to fill 6 x 70cl bottles

4.5 litres birch sap
1kg white caster sugar
200g raisins, chopped
juice of 2 lemons
7g sachet wine yeast

As soon as possible after collecting the sap, bring it to the boil in a large stainless-steel pan and add the sugar. Simmer for 10 minutes, then add the raisins, stir, and pour the whole mixture into a food-grade bucket. Leave to cool for 10 minutes, then add the lemon juice.

Prepare the yeast according to the packet instructions and add it to the sap/raisin mixture once the latter has cooled to blood temperature. Cover the bucket. If you're using a proper wine bucket, there will be a small hole in the lid – cover this with a sheet of tissue paper so that air can get in but insects stay out. Leave for 3 days in a warmish place, by which time the mixture will be fermenting nicely. Strain into a 4.5 litre demijohn and apply an airlock. Leave in a warm, dark place (such as an airing cupboard) until the mixture stops fermenting, then siphon the liquid carefully, leaving the debris (lees) at the bottom. Decant into sterilised bottles, cork, and store in a place with a consistently cool temperature. The wine will be quaffable within 4 weeks, but develops a more rounded flavour after 6 months – you'll have a very delicious wine ready for Christmas.

Calendula

Calendula officinalis

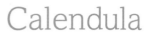

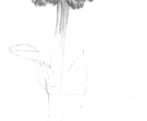

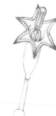

*Showy, orange or yellow,
daisy-like flower heads in
summer and autumn*

Simple, aromatic leaves

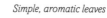

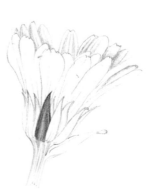

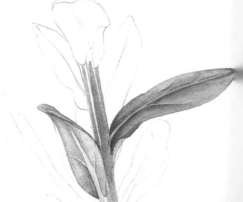

Native to the Mediterranean as well as parts of Asia and southern Europe, calendula marigolds will grow just about anywhere, as an annual in cooler climates and as a hardy shrub elsewhere. The French marigold (known as *Tagetes*) is also edible. The leaves of *Tagetes lucida* are used as a substitute for tarragon; you may see this sold as *pericon* in parts of France and Spain.

The name calendula comes from the Romans, who believed that the flowers bloomed on the first day (the 'calends') of the month. One of the German folk names for the calendula is 'monk's head'. This is because, when the petals have fallen away from the flower head, the remaining seeds look a bit like ... well, the head of a monk. And if you're superstitious, you might be happy to know that a marigold flower popped under your mattress will not only give you dreams of the future, but will also help those dreams come true. So let's hope those dreams are nice ones. Marigold, the name, carries more than a whiff of the Church, originating as 'Mary's Gold', the gift of those who couldn't afford the real thing to give to the Virgin. Calendula means 'little clock' or 'little calendar', possibly because it can bloom all year round. Ancient Greek, Roman, Indian and Middle Eastern civilisations used the flowers as a dye.

Common Names
Pot marigold, ruddles, common marigold, garden marigold, English marigold, Scottish marigold, monk's head.

Medicinal Use
Calendula has been used for centuries, if not millennia, as a medicinal herb. As such, it has a wide range of uses. Externally, it is used as a lotion or ointment on wounds to aid healing (the leaves help the blood to coagulate), as an anti-inflammatory and a sting-soother; latterly it has been used in treating dermatitis and skin problems caused by radiation. Internally, calendula is taken as a tincture for constipation and cramps as well as for dispelling tumours. It is contraindicated in early pregnancy.

Culinary Use
Calendula is still sometimes known as pot marigold. This doesn't refer to the plant pot but to the cooking pot, a testimony to its edibility. Although lots of flowers, technically, are edible, many of them actually taste of close to nothing; the calendula, however, has a good flavour: spicy and slightly nutty, it is actually worth considering as a foodstuff. As well as the petals, the leaves, too, can be eaten, although you'd be unlikely to want to do much more with them apart from adding to soups or cooking as you would

spinach. Add the petals to salads and sandwiches, fold them into fresh ice-cream, whisk then into crème fraiche and use to top sweet crêpes. You can make a tea of the fresh or dried petals, which are sometimes called poor man's saffron because of the colour and slightly spicy flavour they can impart to rice. Try it by stirring two marigold heads' worth of petals into rice pudding. That same pigment can also be used to colour butter and cheese, custards and liqueurs, and is simply extracted from the plant by boiling.

Drying Calendula Petals

The good thing about harvesting and drying the petals is that removing the flowers will encourage more flowers to grow. Pick the flower from its base and then cut the head from the stem. You can use a dehydrator if you have one, but the flowers dry well enough without any help.

Put the flower heads face-down on a sheet of brown paper, on a drying rack or a tray, and leave in a dark, cool place for a few days. The petals should come away from the heads with no effort when they are completely dry – if they don't, leave them for another day or two. Store in an airtight jar (Marmite jars are great for storing herbs because the dense brown glass keeps the light out). The simplest thing to do with the dried petals is to infuse them as a tea. A single teaspoon per cup infused in a transparent glass teapot looks pretty.

Marigold Butterfly Buns

The marigold petals used in these cakes give them a lovely yellow colour.

Makes 18

2 tablespoons fresh marigold petals,
   plus a further tablespoon to garnish
100g self-raising flour
½ teaspoon baking powder
a pinch of ground cloves
100g butter, at room temperature
100g golden caster sugar, plus extra
   for sprinkling
2 medium eggs, lightly beaten
100ml double cream
50g icing sugar

Preheat the oven to 160°C/gas 3. Line an 18-hole fairy cake tin with 18 small fairy-cake cases.

Wash and dry the marigold petals.

Sift the flour together with the baking powder and ground cloves into a bowl and set aside.

In a large mixing bowl, cream together the butter and sugar with a wooden spoon (or use an electric mixer) until fluffy. Add the eggs a little at a time, beating to combine well with each addition and adding a small dredge of the flour mixture with the last bit of egg to stop the mixture from curdling. Add the rest of the flour a little at a time and mix until smooth and silky. Gently fold in 2 tablespoons of marigold petals, then spoon the mixture into the fairy-cake cases.

Bake for about 25 minutes, or until the tops of the cakes are golden brown and an inserted skewer comes out clean. Leave the cakes to cool a little in their tin, then transfer to a wire rack to cool completely. When cooled, carefully slice the top off each cake with a sharp knife, and cut the top in half to make two half-moon shapes.

To make the icing, put the cream in a bowl and sift in the icing sugar. Whip until the cream has stiffened, then stir in the remaining marigold petals.

Ice the top of the fairy cakes and place two butterfly 'wings', made from the pieces of cake that you sliced off, on top of each. Garnish each with a marigold petal.

Pickled Calendula Petals

An interesting dish and likely to be something that any prospective dinner guests won't have eaten before. The petals have to be fresh, so you'll need a decent crop of flowers. If you don't have enough, you can also add any edible petals – roses, dog daisies, violets, nasturtiums, borage and chive. You can also include buds.

Use a clean glass jar, preferably one with a vacuum seal. Measure the volume of the jar – to do this, fill it with water and then pour the water into a marked measuring jug. Make sure that the fresh petals are clean and dry, and half-fill the jar with them. Pour demerara sugar over the petals until the jar is almost full.

Measure out half the jar's volume of white wine vinegar. Pour it into a pan with a few black peppercorns, then bring to the boil and allow to cool. Carefully and gradually pour the spiced vinegar into the jar, allowing the vinegar to be absorbed by the sugar. Seal and leave to mature for 4 days.

This pickle works very well as a slaw or with strong cheeses and meats.

Canna Lily

Canna

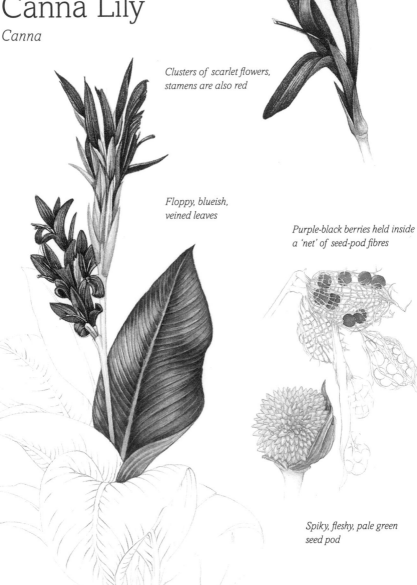

Clusters of scarlet flowers,
stamens are also red

Floppy, blueish,
veined leaves

Purple-black berries held inside
a 'net' of seed-pod fibres

Spiky, fleshy, pale green
seed pod

Canna belongs to the same family as bananas and ginger, as well as *Maranta*, a plant which gives us the thickening agent arrowroot. In Europe, the canna is often grown simply for its beauty, generally without the gardener having any idea that it is edible. The *C. edulis* variety, illustrated here, grows to a height of 1.5m and has a small, exotic-looking reddish-orange flower which resembles a slimmed-down iris blossom. Its cousin, *C. flaccida*, is a little shorter in height, reaching a maximum of 1m, with larger, showier yellow flowers that look even more like an iris. There are a significant number of hybrids, as you'd imagine with such a pretty garden flower. The plant has large, fancy, often-variegated green and purple leaves and it likes to grow with its roots in soggy, marshy ground and its flowers basking in full sun; the dank ditches at the edges of forests prove a good environment. Canna is not frost-resistant, but it grows fast – and despite originally being a native of South America it grows well in northern climates, although you might be advised to uproot the rhizomes and store over harsh winters.

Common Names and Species

Queensland arrowroot, achira, Indian shot, *Canna indica* (the *C. edulis* variety).

Medicinal Use

In Bangladesh, a paste of the plant was used to treat tonsillitis. Research is being carried out into further uses of canna, including whether it could strengthen the body's defences against the Aids virus.

Culinary Use

Cannas have been a common foodstuff for some 4,500 years in the Americas, where they are still used as food for people and as fodder for animals. Where it grows well, the plant is ready to harvest just six months after it is first planted and, because it grows prolifically, it provides an abundant supply. It can be prepared in a variety of ways. The young leaves and shoots have an unusual, sweet-and-sour flavour and can be sautéed in oil or steamed and eaten drizzled with melted butter and a squeeze of lemon juice. The seeds, too, are edible, although they are too tough and hard to be of any use to the casual garden forager. It's the starchy, nutrient-rich rhizomes that are most often served. In Peru they were traditionally cooked in earth ovens: holes were dug in the ground and lined with hot stones, then covered with branches, ash and earth to retain the heat for cooking. The soft, roasted flesh of the canna was then eaten like a baked potato. *C. edulis* has the largest tubers and so is the most popular variety for culinary uses. If a hot-stone earth oven is not an option, the tubers can simply be wrapped in silver foil and cooked in the oven at 200°C/gas 6 in much the same way as a potato. This can take some time, up to 6 hours depending on the thickness of the tuber. Unlike 'normal' potatoes, canna tubers can also be eaten raw – sliced up, like an apple. You can use them raw, too, to provide crunch in salads or sandwiches; slice thinly and use sparingly since they are quite fibrous.

In China and Vietnam, canna is considered too good for animals and is used purely for human consumption. If you've ever eaten Chinese vermicelli – the almost-transparent cellophane noodles – you might be surprised to know that they are made from canna starch. In Australia *Canna edulis* is also known as Queensland arrowroot since the plant makes a similar easily digestible starch.

Chaufa Rice

Serves 6 as a main dish

3½ tablespoons vegetable oil
500g boiled or roasted mixed meats
    (e.g. pork and chicken)
3cm fresh root ginger, grated
3 shallots, chopped
50g canna tubers, peeled and sliced
1kg cooked white rice
1 omelette, made with 3 large eggs,
    and chopped
3 tablespoons soy sauce
salt and pepper, to taste
a handful of young canna shoots,
    to serve (optional)

Heat the oil in a large, heavy-bottomed frying pan over a high heat. Add the meat and grated ginger, stir well and fry until the meat is lightly browned and the ginger is fragrant. Add the shallots and the slices of canna, stir and cook for 2 minutes before adding the rice. Lower the heat and stir the rice so that it covers the bottom of the pan. Add the chopped-up omelette. Continue to cook so that the rice is slightly toasted on the bottom and you have some lovely crispy bits. Add the soy sauce, season with salt and pepper and serve with a few canna shoots topping each bowl, as well some of the delicious crispy rice scraped from the bottom of the pan.

Chinese Dogwood

Cornus kousa var. *chinensis*

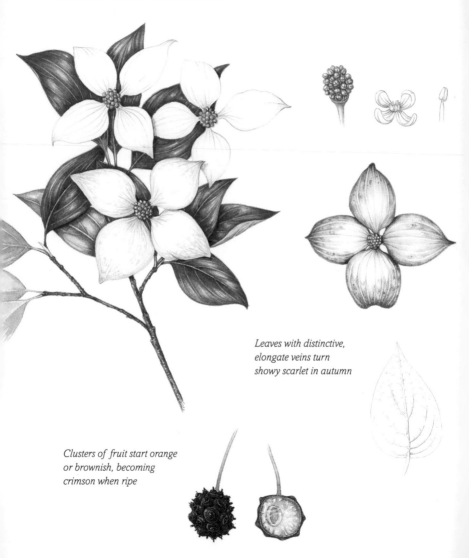

Leaves with distinctive,
elongate veins turn
showy scarlet in autumn

Clusters of fruit start orange
or brownish, becoming
crimson when ripe

A woodland plant and part of the dogwood family, *Cornus kousa* is often grown specifically for its brightly coloured stems that strike a cheerful red or yellow note in the midst of winter. While some dogwoods are evergreen, the *chinensis* variety is deciduous.

Chinese dogwood is also grown for its large, showy bracts, which resemble creamy white or pale pink four-petalled flowers – from a distance, the flat blooms resemble some types of hydrangea. The little greeny-yellow flower in the centre of these bracts is inconspicuous.

A native of East Asia, *Cornus kousa* prefers moist, fertile, well-drained soil, being rather averse to shallow or chalky ground. It's hardy and prefers full sun or partial shade. Left to its own devices, the plant will grow into a sprawling bush up to about 6m high and 5m wide, but in ornamental gardens (where they are often planted) they may well be pruned into a more controlled, elegant shape. In autumn, its leaves are a lovely deep winey-red colour. The abundant fruits start to appear in the autumn and are about the size of a damson, with a knobbly surface, a bit like a lychee, greenish-pink in colour and ripening to a magenta-red hue. For optimum sweetness, wait until they are soft to the touch before harvesting.

Common Names and Species

Kousa, Szechuan strawberry, Korean dogwood, *Benthamidia kousa*, *Cornus mas* (cornelian cherry) also has edible fruits.

Medicinal Use

Some species of dogwood contain pain-killing compounds in their bark and were once used to treat ailments such as headache and toothache. The cornelian cherry *(C. mas)*, which also goes by the name of *zao pi* in China, is used in Chinese herbal medicine to treat a number of ailments including male impotence.

Culinary Use

The *Cornus kousa* fruit is delicious and has a rather exotic flavour, making it one of the most delectable free fruits from an unexpected source. They are lovely eaten raw, with a sweet taste that is a blend of banana, cucumber/melon and strawberry/raspberry with a hint of papaya. The fruit does contain a few seeds, so you should bite through the rather acidic skin and squeeze the fruit to release the yellow/orange flesh, then spit out the seeds in as elegant a way as you can muster. The fruits can also be juiced and used to make jellies and jams.

Chinese-Dogwood Wine

Makes enough to fill 6 x 70cl bottles

1kg ripe Chinese dogwood fruits
4.5 litres boiling water
1kg white caster sugar
juice of 1 lemon
juice of 1 orange
7g sachet wine yeast

Pick over the fruits and wash them thoroughly. Put them into a food-grade plastic bucket and crush with a potato masher – don't worry about skin or pips since all solids will be strained out. Pour the boiling water over them, stir, then cover and leave in a warm place for 3 days, stirring daily.

Strain through a wine bag, discarding the debris (add it to your composter). Put the sugar into the bucket and pour the strained liquid over it. Add the lemon and orange juice and stir well. Make up the yeast according to the packet instructions and add to the liquid. Leave in a warm place (at least 18°C) for 24 hours, by which time the mixture will be starting to ferment. Pour into a fermenting jar and insert an airlock. Leave for up to 4 months; by this time the fermentation should have stopped and there will be a cloudy residue – called 'lees' – at the bottom of the jar. If it's still fermenting, leave it for a little longer.

Siphon the liquid from the lees into another, sterilised demijohn and insert a cork. Leave for a couple of weeks before bottling.

Chinese-Dogwood Posset

Serves 4–6

450g ripe Chinese dogwood fruits
(to make 400ml fruit purée)
900ml double cream
250g white caster sugar
juice of 1 medium lemon

To make the purée, simply remove as many seeds as possible from the fruit and blend until smooth in a food processor or pass the fruit through a fine-meshed sieve.

Put the cream and sugar into a pan and bring to the boil. Remove from the heat, stir in the lemon juice and the fruit purée. Pour into wine glasses and leave to set. Chill in the fridge before serving with biscotti.

Chinese-Dogwood Jam

Makes enough to fill 3 x 340g jars

1kg ripe Chinese dogwood fruits,
chopped into quarters
1kg white granulated sugar
10 cardamom pods, crushed
1 fresh red chilli, finely chopped
1 teaspoon vanilla extract

Wash the fruits and crush them a little in a bowl with a potato masher. Remove as many of the seeds as you can at this stage, but don't worry too much about them.

Put the fruits along with the sugar and cardamom into a heavy-bottomed pan and cook over a low heat to dissolve the sugar. Leave to cool, then strain through a fine-meshed sieve to remove any more seeds and the cardamom pods.

Return the fruit pulp to the pan and add the chilli. If you have one, clip a sugar thermometer to the inside of the pan and bring to the boil over a low heat. Boil until the temperature reaches 105°C, or use the cold saucer method (see page 13) to test if it has reached setting point. Remove the pan from the heat, leave for a couple of minutes, then stir in the vanilla. Pour into warm, sterilised jars and, when completely cold, cover with waxed discs and put on the lids.

Chokeberry

Aronia melanocarpa

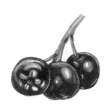

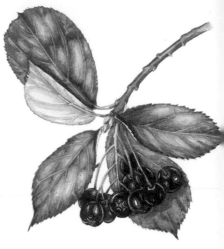

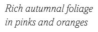

*Rich autumnal foliage
in pinks and oranges*

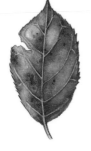

*Very shiny, prolific, black-purple
fruit hangs in clusters*

*Showy, pale pink or white blossom
with little hawthorn-like petals*

Aronia is a medium-sized shrub whose leaves start to turn a beautiful, brilliant flame colour from late summer onwards, brightening up gardens, as do the berries, which range from red (*A. arbutifolia*) to black (*A. melanocarpa*) or a shade somewhere between the two, a sort of purplish-black (*A. x prunifolia*). In the spring, pale pink and white blossoms precede the berries. Native to northeast America and now naturalised all over Europe, chokeberries are tough and versatile plants, hardy and frost-resistant, happy to lodge themselves even in wooded areas of poor or acidic soil and preferring a damp environment. In Poland the plants are grown to produce a tea, and in Lithuania to make a wine. Here in the UK, innovative growers in Wales are planting crops of chokeberries to make an exclusive liqueur called Aerona, and Marks and Spencer are so excited about chokeberries that they're cultivating them in Scotland as part of a plan to popularise the fruits, although the shrubs themselves have been well established in many UK gardens for decades. The berries of all three varieties are not only edible but now heralded as a superfood, although its popular name chokeberry is a bit of a giveaway, as the berries are tongue-curlingly sour if eaten raw (chokeberry extract is an ingredient in Haribo Tangfastics).

Common Species and Cultivars
A. arbutifolia, A. x prunifolia.

Medicinal Use
The fruits of the chokeberry are even richer in antioxidants than the better-known acai and goji berries and contain 15 times more vitamin C than the blueberry; indeed they've been described as the 'healthiest fruit in the world' and have the highest-ever recorded concentration of anthocyanins (powerful antioxidants, important in fighting cancer and other illnesses) of any berry. Not only that, but Native Americans regarded the berries as a powerful aphrodisiac. Otherwise, the use of aronia in fighting cancer is currently being studied independently. Clipper make a herbal tea – Organic Red Fruits and Aronia Berry – and you can buy aronia supplements from health-food outlets; among the claims made by their manufacturers is their effectiveness in reducing oxidative stress, a phenomenon linked to many chronic illnesses such as heart disease.

Culinary Use
Various aronia products, including tinctures, juices and the dried berries, can be bought, generally from health-food outlets, but at a premium. So, if you have an established aronia bush in your garden, it's well worth harvesting your own berries. And if you

don't have one, you might want to consider buying one as an investment in a healthy future. They grow quickly, can be cultivated from cuttings and a decent-sized pot from a garden centre will cost less than the price of a bottle of the juice or a pack of the dried berries. Aronia, like most berries, is best harvested before the first frost.

Because the fruits don't contain stones or pips, they're ideal for making jams, jellies and sauces or blending with other fruits to make smoothies.

If you have an abundant crop, the aronia berries can be juiced or made into a sauce, in much the same way as cranberries, in order to preserve them for use in other recipes. Freeze the berries first in order to soften the skins.

Aronia-Berry Cordial

Makes approx. 500ml

*500g ripe aronia berries (a mix of
    berries from different species, if
    you're lucky enough to have access
    to them)*
200g white caster sugar, or more to taste
juice of 1 lemon

Put the berries into a pan and cover with water. Cover the pan and place over a low heat for about 15 minutes or until the berries are soft. Drain the berries, reserving the cooking liquid. Push the berries through a fine-meshed sieve to reserve any pulp while getting rid of the pips.

Put the juice and pulp back into the pan along with the sugar and lemon juice. Heat gently, stirring, until the sugar is dissolved. Decant immediately into warm, sterilised jars or other containers and store in the fridge; otherwise leave to cool and pour into plastic bottles. Leave a few centimetres at the top to allow for expansion, and freeze.

Dilute with water to taste for a cordial drink. This is also good poured over ice-cream or reduced and thickened to a syrup and used as a glaze for roast meats.

Jane's Aronia Layer Cake

Serves 8–10

For the sponge
320g self-raising flour
50g cocoa powder
2 teaspoons bicarbonate of soda
300g white caster sugar
300g butter, at room temperature
4 eggs, beaten
100ml full-fat milk
100ml aronia cordial, see opposite
150g beetroot, boiled and finely grated

For the cream filling
100g butter
140g icing sugar, sifted, plus extra for
the top of the cake
100g crème fraiche
100g mascarpone

Preheat the oven to 180°C/gas 4. Grease two 20cm cake tins and line with baking parchment.

To make the sponge, sift the flour and cocoa powder into a bowl or food processor and add all the other ingredients except for the beetroot. Mix until smooth, then fold in the grated beetroot and stir to combine well.

Spoon the mixture into the prepared tins and bake for 50–60 minutes or until an inserted skewer comes out clean. Turn the tins halfway through the baking time to ensure the cakes cook evenly.

To make the filling, beat together the butter and icing sugar until fluffy. Spread on top of one of the cakes. Then beat together the crème fraiche and mascarpone and spread over the butter and icing-sugar mix. Layer the second cake on top and lightly dust the top of the cake with icing sugar.

Dahlia

Dahlia

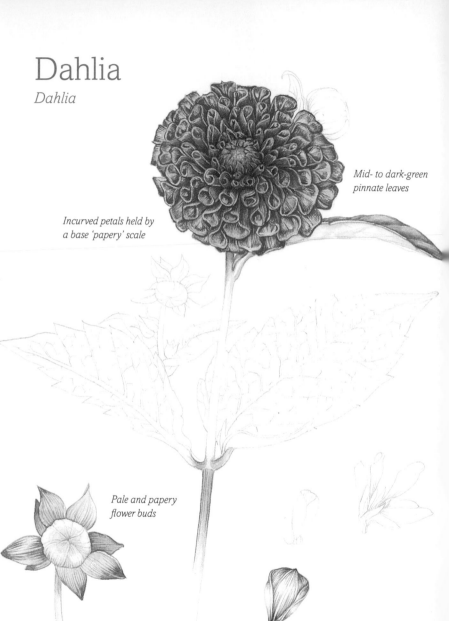

Mid- to dark-green
pinnate leaves

Incurved petals held by
a base 'papery' scale

Pale and papery
flower buds

The dahlia is the national flower of Mexico, where it originated as a wild flower. There are now over 30 recognised species and at least 20,000 cultivars of the plant. When it first arrived in Europe in the 18th century, the flower became a great favourite not only of Marie Antoinette but also of Josephine Bonaparte and by the middle of the 19th century there was full-blown dahlia fever, with keen gardeners competing with one another to create bigger and bigger and more and more colourful blooms. The flowers themselves are not dissimilar to those of certain sunflower cultivars, so it won't come as a surprise to find that the two are related, as they are to dandelions, marigolds, daisies and chrysanthemums, too. In the case of the *Dahlia imperialis*, the plant grows taller than many trees, up to 7m, although the flowers themselves are relatively small. The Mexicans called the tall, hollow-stemmed tree dahlia *chichipatl*, meaning 'cane flower', or *acacotli*, meaning 'water cane'. The stems carry a large amount of water and consequently must have been a welcome sight to the Mexicans. The tubers, too, are extremely juicy; unfortunately, it's this high water content which also makes dahlias susceptible to frost, and if they're to survive the winter in less temperate climes, the tubers have to be uprooted and kept indoors.

Medicinal Use

A naturally occurring fruit sugar called inulin (or dahlin) can be extracted from the plant and was used in the treatment of diabetes before the discovery of insulin. Some tribes used the petals, crushed up, as a means of soothing insect bites and stings.

Culinary Use

These showy garden flowers, whose prim starbursts of petals have been a stalwart of many a village fete, flower show or arrangement, have recently been discovered by a whole new audience of foodies.

Although dahlia petals are edible, they're nothing to write home about, to be honest. Where the dahlia comes into its own in the kitchen is with its tubers. We're really only just discovering the tasty tubers in the west thanks, in part, to the gardener James Wong drawing our attention to them in newspaper articles and on the TV, but dahlia tubers have been a traditional food in Central America for centuries, particularly in the mountains of southern Mexico; in fact, when the plant was introduced to Europe it was not only for its decorative properties but also as a root vegetable. The Swedish botanist Andreas Dahl, after whom they were named, tried to popularise them as an alternative to the humble spud.

If you'd like to try growing dahlias specifically for their flavour, try some of the older varieties that were around before we started breeding them purely for show; 'Yellow Gem' is a good one to hunt out, as are 'Lemon Chiffon' and 'Inland Dynasty'. You'll notice that the older varieties have more abundant tubers, too, since of course this is what the original cultivators were interested in.

The flavour of a dahlia tuber is not dissimilar to that of a Jerusalem artichoke (the two plants are related) and they can be used in the same way as a potato, but in truth it's unlikely that any of us are actually going to cook a huge load of the tubers and mash them with butter … not just yet, anyway. The crunchy texture (a bit like radishes or water chestnuts) and delicate flavour lends itself well to the fragrant spices associated with Asian dishes and they make a good substitute for water chestnuts.

As with any root vegetable, wash the tubers thoroughly. It's not always necessary to peel them if you want to roast them in the oven with olive oil and garlic, but do try the tuber first before you cook it, to see if you like it. If you're going to enjoy this interesting vegetable raw, in a salad for example, then it's better peeled and thinly sliced. If you don't like the flavour, pot it up and enjoy as a flower.

Dahlia-Tuber Stir-Fry

Serves 3–4

125g dahlia tuber
2 tablespoons sunflower or vegetable oil
225g beansprouts
1 carrot, cut into 4cm batons
1 garlic clove, crushed
3cm fresh root ginger, finely grated
2 spring onions, chopped on the slant
salt and pepper, to taste
2 teaspoons sesame oil
2 tablespoons soy sauce

For the garnish
125g cashew nuts
1 lime, cut into 4 wedges
a handful of fresh coriander, chopped
a sprinkle of fresh green coriander seeds
  (optional)

Peel the dahlia tuber and slice it thinly, then blot with kitchen paper to remove excess juice.

Dry-toast the cashew nuts (for the garnish) in a wok, shaking them constantly so that they don't scorch. Remove from the pan and set aside.

Add the sunfower or vegetable oil to the wok and heat. Add the beansprouts, sliced dahlia tuber, carrot, garlic, ginger and spring onions, then season well with salt and pepper and cook over a medium to high heat for about 5 minutes, stirring all the time. Stir in the sesame oil and soy sauce and cook for a further minute.

Serve in bowls on top of rice or noodles, garnished with the toasted cashew nuts, the lime wedges, chopped coriander and a sprinkle of green coriander seeds (if using).

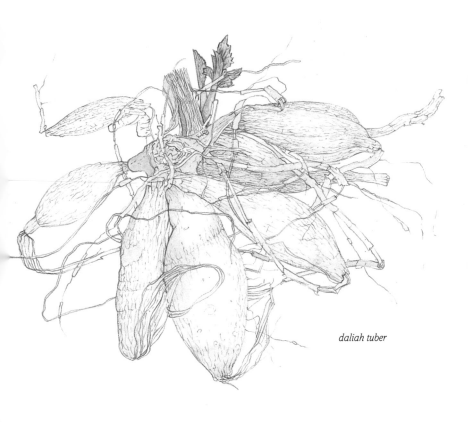

daliah tuber

Day Lily
Hemerocallis fulva

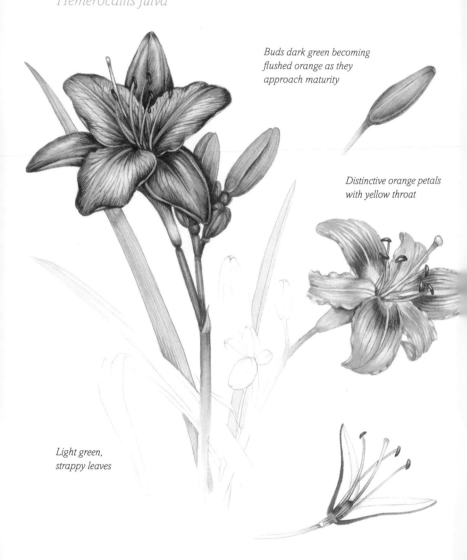

Buds dark green becoming
flushed orange as they
approach maturity

Distinctive orange petals
with yellow throat

Light green,
strappy leaves

The name of this plant comes from the Greek *hemera*, meaning 'day', and *kalos*, meaning 'beautiful', an accurate description of this pretty flower which, alas, has a life of only 24 hours. However, it's not all bad news. The blossom that was fresh in the morning might be a sad heap of withered petals by night-time, but a new flower blooms again in place of the old one the next day. So, while day lilies may disappoint if used in formal flower arrangements, they make up for this by being a wonderfully prolific garden flower. So prolific, in fact, that they can become invasive, which makes it the perfect edible garden plant.

The day lily has been hybridised to come in a range of different colours, most commonly a tawny-orange. Reaching no higher than 1m, it has light green, strappy leaves and stems that bear bundles of different-sized, tight green elongated flower buds. The plant is a hardy perennial and, in the right conditions, will keep its leaves all year round. Day lilies prefer sunny conditions and moist (slightly soggy) fertile soil and will happily colonise patches of ground, spreading by means of underground rhizomes, sometimes to the point of being regarded as a pest despite their beauty. Depending on the climate, blossoming time can be any time between the beginning of spring to early autumn. There are many different day lilies; over 72,000 are listed on the database of the American Hemerocallis Society. However, it's the *Hemerocallis fulva* variety we are most interested in here. It originated in Asia, where it has been grown as a foodstuff since time immemorial. Arguably this most common day lily had reached Europe by the 15th century via the Silk Routes and was introduced to America by the early European settlers. We don't know for certain if all day-lily species and cultivars are edible, but *H. graminea* is also fine and likely to be the one you might find on the menu if you happen to be travelling in Asia. ('Graminea' means 'stiff grass' and refers to the leaves of the plant).

Medicinal Use

The Roman philosopher Pliny the Elder advised that day-lily tea would ease the pain of childbirth; indeed, the flower was used up until the 19th century as a painkiller, made into a simple infusion of fresh blossom, hot water and honey and taken either internally (for headaches) or else used to soak bandages which were then applied to sprains and aching muscles. More recent studies have confirmed that it does indeed contain analgesic properties, as well as a significant amount of antioxidants, although specific research into its pain-killing qualities has yet to take place. Day-lily tea was once used as a gargle to soothe toothache. In China, the word for the flower is synonymous with the meaning to 'forget worry', hence the plant is also believed to lift the spirits, though this might just as well refer to the prettiness of the flowers as anything else.

Culinary Use

Flavour-wise the young buds have a satisfying kick, a bit like green beans with a hint of the sharpness of radish or onion. The fresh flower petals, too, have a sweet taste and a grainy texture, and the tubers – the best part for most day-lily aficionados – are starchy and sweetly nutty, rather like a sweet potato except, sometimes, with a slight hint of acid, reminiscent of a sharp apple. They have a juicy, slippery texture. The stems are also edible but not especially appetising.

There are a variety of ways you can use day lilies in the kitchen. The flower petals can be dried, crumbled and used, like saffron, to colour rice. Fresh petals can be infused to make a tea, as mentioned above – remove any green bits at the base of the petal as they taste bitter and will mar the delicate sweetness of the petal itself. The stamens and pistils don't taste so great, so remove them too. The fresh flowers themselves can be covered in tempura batter and deep-fried, or served stuffed with ice-cream or sorbet for an easy but exotic-looking desert.

Day-lily buds are a classic ingredient in certain Chinese and Asian dishes, including hot-and-sour soups and pork dishes, and you can find them in Asian supermarkets, packaged as Golden Needles, Gum Jum or just plain Lily Buds.

The fresh buds (which give a good burst of vitamin A as well as iron) are delicious sautéed in a little butter with a squeeze of lemon or lime, as a side dish. They are also good eaten raw, which is the best way to try them to get a clear idea of the flavour. Eat only the smaller, younger buds, though – once over 12cm in length they are inclined to be tough.

If you want to try the tubers, they are at their best in early spring or late summer when they will be white and tender (if they're old and brown, don't bother) and have a lovely fresh nutty taste. If you dig up the plant, you'll see a tangle of roots ending in elongated torpedo-shaped tubers. Snip off half of the tubers and put the plant back in the ground. Remove any fine root hairs and wash thoroughly, using a vegetable brush, then cook in the same way as potatoes – boiled, steamed or roasted.

Day-Lily Ice-Cream

Makes 6–8 generous helpings

8 fresh day-lily flowers
1 litre single cream
125ml double cream
150g golden caster sugar
2 teaspoons vanilla extract

Prepare the day-lily flowers by removing any green bits at the base of the petal. Remove the stamens and pistils too.

Mix the flowers with all the remaining ingredients in a bowl and churn the ice-cream in an ice-cream maker, following the manufacturer's instructions. Alternatively, put the mixture into a clean freezer container and freeze for about 1 hour or until almost frozen, then stir thoroughly with a fork to break up the crystals and return to the freezer. Remove from the freezer 15 minutes before serving.

Douglas Fir
Pseudotsuga menziesii

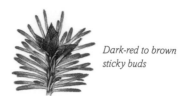

Dark-red to brown
sticky buds

Under side of each needle
is pale and silvery

Younger tips are
brighter green and soft

Distinctively fringed cones

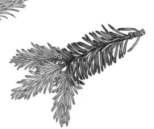

Although the Douglas fir is seldom found growing in small gardens, a walk through any forested area of pine trees will surely yield a stand of Douglas firs at some point. But there's an even easier way to access a Douglas fir as a domesticated plant. If you happen to be buying a rooted Christmas tree, pay a little extra and invest in an organically grown Douglas fir. Over the holiday period keep it well watered, then in January plant it out where it will be able to grow properly, and return every year to harvest some of the fir tips for use in the kitchen. Careful where you plant it, though; Douglas firs can grow incredibly tall. The tallest one on record in the UK is currently 64m high, a mere dwarf in comparison with a tree reputed to be 126m high, cut down in Vancouver in 1902, or an even taller specimen which hit the ground a couple of years earlier after growing to an astonishing 142m. Bear in mind when planting, too, that your little potted tree can live for more than a thousand years. Despite originating in the US, the Douglas fir is naturalised in Europe.

Common Names
Oregon pine or Oregon spruce.

Medicinal Use
Although Douglas fir is not often used as a medicine these days, Native Americans used it in a variety of ways; the resin, which has antiseptic properties, was applied as a poultice to cuts and burns. The resin was also chewed to soothe sore throats. An infusion of the young twigs and shoots was used as a remedy for ailments of the bladder and kidneys. If you're a runner or a jogger, try placing the young fresh sprigs in the tips of your trainers to stop your feet from sweating and to prevent athlete's foot.

Culinary Use
It's a little-known fact that the young tips of all pine trees are edible and you could certainly substitute the Douglas-fir needles and tips with whatever pine you have in your garden or nearby; don't get confused with other evergreens such as leylandii, though, as these are not edible. Pick the pine tips just as they first start to appear; the young tips look like pale green tufts at the ends of the boughs. Remove any of the brown papery casings. Different trees produce slightly different tastes but the words you'll find yourself using are lemony, resiny and, unsurprisingly, piney! The flavour gets sweeter with cooking. Be aware, though, that when you pick the tips you restrict growth to that branch for that year.

Pine-Infused Sugar

This simple, flavoured sugar is a nice and easy way to start experimenting with pine in the kitchen.

Weigh equal volumes of fresh, young fir tips and granulated sugar. Place in a food processor and pulse in short bursts, until finely ground and powder-like, then spread on a tray to dry completely – there's a surprising amount of moisture in those tips. If lumps form, break them up with a fork. When the tips are dry, after a day or so, store them in an airtight jar. The resulting fine powder tastes lovely and lends an appropriately festive taste sprinkled over warm mince pies. You might also try adding dried, ground spruce tips to shop-bought mayonnaise to give an exciting twist to sandwiches or even for dipping your chips into!

Fir-Tip Syrup

Makes approx. 75cl

400g golden caster sugar
500ml water
200g young fir/spruce tips, washed
  and roughly chopped

Put all the ingredients into a heavy-bottomed pan over a medium heat and bring to the boil. Reduce the heat, cover and simmer for about 5 minutes. Remove from the heat and leave to cool. Strain the syrup through a fine-meshed sieve into a warm, sterilised jar and discard the fir tips. Store in a bottle in the refrigerator. Pour over pancakes or waffles, or stir into plain yoghurt.

Fir-Tip Shortbread

Makes 20–25 biscuits

325g plain flour
200g unsalted butter, chilled and
 cut into small cubes
125g golden caster sugar
4 tablespoons finely chopped fir tips,
 washed
2 large egg yolks, beaten
icing sugar, for dusting

Sift the flour into a bowl and rub in the butter until the mixture resembles fresh breadcrumbs. Add the caster sugar and the fir tips and mix thoroughly to combine, then mix in the beaten yolks. Knead lightly to form a dough with a pretty green tint. Put the dough in a plastic freezer bag and refrigerate for about half an hour.

Preheat the oven to 160°C/gas 3. Line a 20 x 30cm baking tray with greaseproof paper and dust the paper with icing sugar.

Form the dough into 20–25 balls and press each one on to the lined baking tray to make a disc about 1.5–2cm thick. Lightly score each shortbread biscuit with a fork. Bake for 5 minutes, then turn down the oven to 150°C/gas 2. Bake for a further 15–20 minutes – the biscuits should be a light golden brown. Remove from the oven and leave to cool on the tray.

Fir-Tip Tipple

Try this for a sensational Christmas Eve tipple!

Makes 350ml

Pound 2 tablespoons of spruce or pine needles in a mortar to release their wonderful scent. Add them to a 350ml bottle of gin or vodka along with 1 tablespoon of white sugar. Leave to infuse overnight, then strain the spirit and discard the ground pine needles. Decant the vodka or gin back into its bottle – it will have turned a lovely pale pistachio colour and tastes great served on its own over ice or with added tonic or soda water.

Fiddlehead Fern

Matteuccia struthiopteris

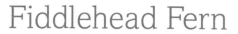

Leaflets vary from watery yellow-green to solid mid-green in colour

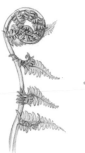

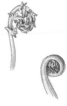

Pale green stems with brownish, papery scales

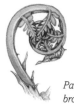

Grows in elongate plumes from central root

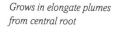

The fiddlehead fern is very aptly named as the young shoots, uncurling delicately from the spring soils, look exactly like the head of a fiddle. The plant is often referred to as a crozier and, for reasons less obvious, also as shuttlecock fern and ostrich fern because the plumy leaves look like ostrich feathers.

This is a popular foraged wild plant in the northern part of the US and is so well known there that it can be bought in farmers' markets. Although it occurs naturally as a wild plant in most parts of northern Europe and across Asia, it isn't as widely recognised in Europe as it is in the US, or in Japan where it is called *kogomi* and is considered a real delicacy. In the UK it is widely available in garden centres and nurseries as a very popular and pretty cultivated plant which is very easy to grow. The fiddlehead fern grows up to 170cm high, with a sprawling habit as it propagates by sending out shoots. It is deciduous, so when planting bear in mind that although the plant looks lovely when in leaf, in the winter months you'll be left with a brown stump after the leaves die back. Also, although its spread is slow, it is inexorable ... so give it some space. Like most ferns, *struthiopteris* likes damp, semi-shaded spaces with rich, sandy soil.

Common Names
Shuttlecock fern, ostrich fern.

Medicinal Use
In folk medicine, fiddleheads are often used as a spring tonic because they appear in the spring, and consuming any fresh green leaves after the stodgy foods of winter is a good thing. They're also infused as a tea and used as a throat gargle. We also know that fiddleheads are rich in omega 3 and omega 6 fatty acids and have plenty of iron and fibre.

Culinary Use
While there are several different edible ferns, such as maidenhair, fiddleheads are one of the most delicious. It's tricky to describe what they taste like, but the young shoots are a bit nutty, a bit grassy, a bit mushroomy and a little bit artichokey. Fiddleheads need to be cooked before eating because there's a slim chance they could give you an upset stomach if eaten raw, and they should be rinsed thoroughly in running water before cooking, to remove any grit. Lightly steamed, sautéed with lemon juice and served with a béarnaise sauce, they taste sensational and look beautiful on the plate, too. The season for them is short, only three to four weeks before the plant has erupted from tight coils to exuberant feathery fronds. Pick the coiled ends with

3–5cm of stem and cook and eat them as soon as possible after picking. Pickling is a good way to preserve them and, again, they look lovely packed in jars.

Fiddlehead Pickle

Makes enough to fill 2 x 250ml jars (or 1 x 500ml jar)

300g fresh young fiddlehead tops
2 tablespoons water
300ml cider vinegar
sea salt, to taste
3 garlic cloves, cut into slivers
1 teaspoon red peppercorns
½ teaspoon mustard seeds
½ teaspoon celery seeds
½ teaspoon cumin seeds

Wash the fiddleheads thoroughly and trim away any brown bits.

Put the water, vinegar and a little sea salt into a non-reactive pan and bring to the boil.

Add the ferns, then cover and cook at a brisk simmer for about 10 minutes.

While the fiddleheads are cooking, divide all the other ingredients between two 250ml jars (or one 500ml jar).

Drain the fiddleheads, reserving their cooking liquid, and leave to cool, then divide between each warm, sterilised jar.

Heat the cooking liquid to boiling point in a small pan and pour over the contents in the jars. Put the lids on the jars and invert them a few times to mix the contents evenly. If necessary, top up with extra vinegar (it doesn't matter if this is cold) so that the fiddleheads are completely immersed.

Remove the lids from the jars and leave the pickle to cool completely. Replace the lids and allow the pickle to mature for a couple of weeks before using.

This is good served with cold meats, oily fish or cheeses.

Firethorn

Pyracantha

*Pale yellow flesh and five
seeds in star-form within
each pome*

*Clusters of
red-orange berries*

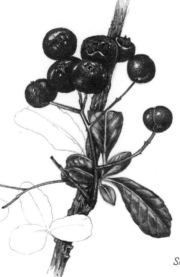

Shiny, serrated leaves

Firethorn is native to a large area spanning Spain, Iran, China and Taiwan. Its spiny thickness makes the shrub a good choice for a secure boundary hedge and you'll also often see it trained against a wall, presumably to stop would-be intruders scaling up it. The pyracantha is generally trimmed back as a garden plant, but left to its own devices it will send its spiky tangle of branches shooting up to 6m tall and to about the same in width. Pyracantha doesn't mind what sort of soil it's planted in, but does prefer sunshine over shade. The pretty panicles of white blossoms, which cover the plant in late spring, are attractive to bees and other insects. The berries that replace the flowers in the autumn range from a yellowish colour through to flame-red and provide welcome food for blackbirds throughout the winter. If you've ever read *The Thorn Birds* by Colleen McCullough, you might remember the story of the mythological birds, which, pierced with the sharpest thorn of the pyracantha, sang a sweeter song than any other bird.

It's easy to confuse the pyracantha with the berberis. *Berberis darwinii* has spikier leaves, a bit like small holly leaves, whereas those of the pyracantha are smooth oval shapes. Also, the pyracantha flowers grow in panicles, while the berberis flowers grow along the length of the stem.

Common Names and Species

Firebush and, more unusually, flameberry, *Pyracantha coccinea*.

Culinary Use

Strictly speaking, pyracantha berries aren't actually berries, but pomes: a fleshy fruit with seeds at the core, like apples (hence 'pomes' from *pommes*). The berries of all varieties are edible, but the taste varies from species to species, so the only way to find out what they taste like is to eat them. Some will have a mild taste and others may be tart, but all have a slightly granular, mealy texture, a bit like a pear. Although they would be slightly toxic if you were to eat a lot of them raw, once they are cooked, they are fine for consumption and with the easy abundance of the berries it's worth giving them a try. Pick the berries when they are bright red, in late autumn – wear gloves to protect your hands. You'll find lots of recipes for pyracantha jams and jellies, and the jelly overleaf, which also contains crab apples (in season at the same time and equally abundant), is one of the nicest I've tried. I also came up with a recipe for a sauce made in the same way as hawthorn-berry ketchup or pontack.

Flameberry Chilli Jelly

Makes enough to fill 3 x 450g jars

1.5kg pyracantha berries
200g crab apples, chopped
1.5kg preserving sugar per 850ml
   strained juice (see method)
1 fresh lemon per 850ml strained juice
1 fresh red chilli per 850ml strained juice

Pick over the berries and wash them thoroughly. Put them in a large heavy-bottomed pan with the chopped apples and cover with 2cm of boiling water. Bring back to the boil and let simmer for 20 minutes.

Leave to cool for about 20 minutes, then strain the juice through a jelly bag into a large bowl for several hours, or preferably overnight. The pulp won't be very appetising to humans, but freeze it and add to the bird table in the winter months.

Measure the strained juice and put in a large, heavy-bottomed pan. For every 850ml of juice, add 1.5kg preserving sugar, the juice of 1 lemon and 1 fresh red chilli, chopped into small pieces. If using a sugar thermometer, place it in the pan with the ingredients.

Bring to the boil, stirring, and skim away any foam that forms on the surface, using a metal spoon. If you have a sugar thermometer, the setting point for jelly is 105°C; otherwise, use the cold saucer test (see page 13). Stir once more to distribute the chopped chillies evenly.

Pour into warm, sterilised jars and, when completely cold, seal with waxed discs and put on the lids.

Flameberry Pontack

Traditionally made with elderberries, pontack is a sauce often served with game, although its rich, fruity, vinegary flavour makes it a great ingredient to add to soups and stews – or to a Bloody Mary instead of Worcestershire sauce. Pyracantha berries lend themselves to the same treatment, although the sauce is best when left for up to a year to mature.

Makes 350ml

650g pyracantha berries
200g golden caster sugar
180ml cider vinegar
450ml water
5 cloves
2 star anise
1 small nutmeg, freshly grated
3cm fresh root ginger, grated
6 shallots, roughly chopped
a pinch of salt

Pick over the berries, remove and discard the stalks, then wash the berries and set aside.

Pour the sugar and cider vinegar into a pan and heat gently until the sugar has completely dissolved. Turn up the heat and boil for 5 minutes before adding the water, berries, spices, shallots and a pinch of salt. Cover and simmer over a low heat for about 1 hour. Set aside and leave to cool.

Strain the sauce through a fine-meshed sieve, scraping the pulp from the underside of the sieve from time to time. Discard the pulp, then return the sauce to the pan and simmer to reduce it by approximately a third. Leave to cool, then pour into sterilised jars and seal the jars.

Fish Weed

Houttuynia cordata

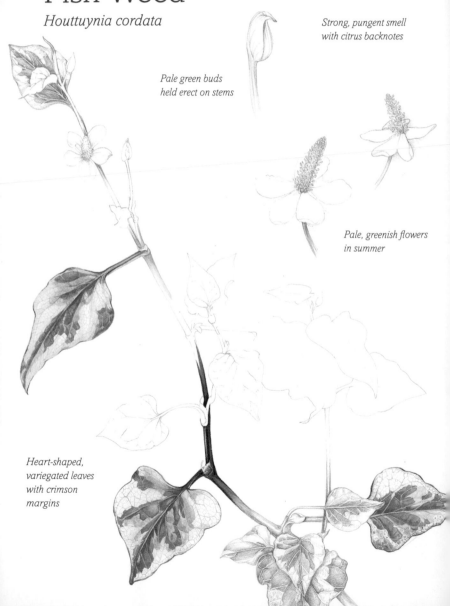

Strong, pungent smell
with citrus backnotes

Pale green buds
held erect on stems

Pale, greenish flowers
in summer

Heart-shaped,
variegated leaves
with crimson
margins

Although this plant originates in East Asia and is native to many regions including Thailand, Vietnam, Nepal and China, it has adapted very well to conditions in the west, too. It is prevalent in the US and Europe, primarily as an ornamental rather than an edible garden plant. Growing to between 20 and 80cm high, the plant has heart-shaped leaves, sometimes variegated, and pretty pale greenish flowers which appear in the summer months. The leaves are used to flavour all sorts of dishes, including curries, and the roots are also used like a vegetable.

If you decide to grow this plant in your garden, be aware that it can be VERY invasive so it is best grown in a large pot or a tub. The fish weed favours full sun or partial shade and a damp soil; the plant will happily thrive with its roots immersed in water. I have a *Houttuynia cordata* 'Chameleon' in my garden in Wales and very beautiful it is, too; the leaves start out as green and gradually develop a lovely pink colour which spreads down from the tip, leaving the bottom part of the leaf green.

Common Names

Fish mint, Vietnamese mint, *diep ca* (Vietnam), chameleon plant, Chinese lizard tail, heartleaf, fishwort, *dokudami* (Japanese for 'poison-blocking plant'), *toningok* (India).

Medicinal Use

During the 2002/2003 outbreak of SARS (severe acute respiratory syndrome), a virus which triggered the deaths of nearly 800 people, mainly in Hong Kong, *Houttuynia* supplements were used to treat symptoms of the disease, and it has been used for generations as a folk remedy against asthma. Otherwise, it is used as a diuretic and detoxifying aid in both Chinese and Japanese complementary therapies.

Culinary Use

Chinese *Houttuynia* leaves have a scent and flavour somewhat akin to coriander, whereas the Japanese variety has a citrusy perfume. As you'd guess from its many folk names, the leaves also add an unmistakable flavour and smell of fish to any dish, so *Houttuynia* doesn't really lend itself to use in desserts. And if you're not keen on fish, it's probably not going to be to your taste – the Chinese name, *vuxing cau*, translates as 'fish stinking herb'. You have been warned!

Asian Spring Rolls with *Houttuynia* Leaves

Makes 15 rolls

70g dried mushrooms (porcini are
  fine and readily available)
70ml (approx.) boiling water
100g clear noodles
90ml (approx.) vegetable oil
2 tablespoons soy sauce
2 tablespoons oyster sauce or
  sushi vinegar
3–4 garlic cloves, finely chopped
2cm fresh root ginger, finely grated
1 small fresh red chilli, finely chopped
  (optional)
2 spring onions, finely chopped
salt and freshly ground pepper, to taste
15 spring-roll wrappers
a good handful of Houttuynia *leaves,*
  finely shredded

Put the mushrooms in a bowl and cover with about 70ml boiling water. Leave to soak for 2 hours. Drain and reserve their soaking water. Blot the soaked mushrooms on some kitchen paper, then slice them thinly.

Cook the noodles according to the packet instructions, then drain and chop into 2cm lengths.

In a heavy-bottomed wok (or frying pan), over a medium heat, heat a little of the oil and, when hot, add the mushrooms, soy sauce and oyster sauce or vinegar. Cook for a minute or so, then turn up the heat, and cook for about 2 minutes or until the mushrooms are soft, adding about 4 tablespoons of the reserved mushroom water as needed – the mixture needs to be on the dry side.

Remove the mushrooms from the wok, and set aside. Put the garlic, ginger and chilli into the wok with a little oil and cook quickly, making sure they don't burn, then add the spring onions and season to taste. Stir-fry for a further minute then remove from the heat and set aside to cool.

To assemble the spring rolls, place the first spring-roll wrapper on a chopping board with a corner facing you. Wet the edges with a little water, using your finger or a pastry brush. Spoon about 2 tablespoonfuls of filling near the bottom corner, then scatter some of the shredded *Houttuynia* leaves over the filling. Roll for one 'turn', tuck in the sides and continue rolling, sealing the roll at the top by brushing with more water if necessary. Repeat with the rest of the rolls and the filling.

Pour the rest of the oil into the wok, heat and fry the spring rolls in batches for about 3–5 minutes until golden brown, then, using a slotted spoon, transfer them to a plate lined with kitchen paper to blot up excess oil and keep them warm.

Serve with rice and a spicy dipping sauce.

Fuchsia

Fuchsia

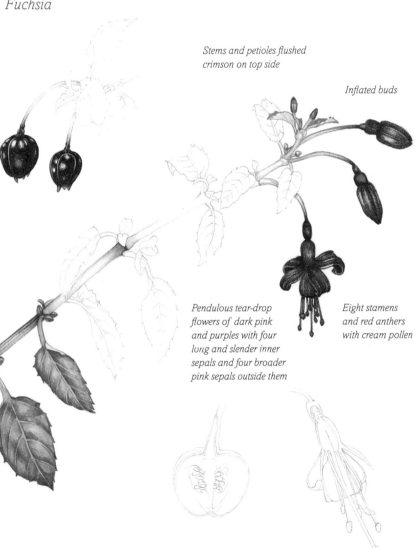

Stems and petioles flushed
crimson on top side

Inflated buds

Pendulous tear-drop
flowers of dark pink
and purples with four
long and slender inner
sepals and four broader
pink sepals outside them

Eight stamens
and red anthers
with cream pollen

It might come as a surprise to many gardeners that the berries which are usually left to rot on their fuchsia plants and shrubs are edible. There are many, many different varieties of fuchsia and while the good news is that all berries of any species can be eaten, the bad news is that edible does not always mean that they are all equally delicious. But then there are many different types of apple, too, and each of us has our own preference – sweet, tart, juicy, dry and everything in between. An additional bonus is that fuchsia flowers are also good to eat, although you'll need to wash them carefully to make sure that any bugs escape from the nooks and crannies in the folds of the petals. The innermost petals are generally softer and sweeter than the outer ones, and the earlier in the season, the more tender the texture.

The majority of fuchsia berries have a good taste. The flavours range from sharp and peppery (which will make a delicious chutney, lovely with meat or cheese) to delicately sweet, which would suit a jam, a jelly or even a pie. There's a general rule of thumb which says 'the blacker the berry, the sweeter the taste'. The *F. procumbens* (a creeping variety) is one of the sweeter types.

Native to South America and discovered in the 17th century in the Caribbean by the French plant collector Plumier, the fuchsia is named after an earlier, German botanist, Leonart Fuchs, whom Plumier admired. (If you have trouble spelling 'fuchsia', bear in mind the German word for 'fox' which it is named after: 'fuchs-ia'. There are over 100 species of the plant, whose dainty, ballerina-like flowers, dangling from the bushes like toys on a Christmas tree, now grace gardens all over the world. Ones that are guaranteed to be winter-hardy in northern climes include *F. magellanica*, illustrated here, which is happy growing at the fringes of woodland; they're the ones with small, narrow, delicate dark red flowers. Fuchsias like a good, well-drained and fertile soil, with their heads partially shaded from the sun and protected against potential frost pockets. In the right conditions, they can grow into shrubs of up to 3m in both height and width.

Medicinal Use

As a folk medicine, fuchsia berries are used to reduce fevers and as a diuretic. Some practitioners of vibrational flower remedies believe that fuchsia helps people accept the grief of past events, enabling them to move forward.

Culinary Use

Most fuchsia berries appear, like other fruits, towards the end of the summer and into the autumn months. They're about the size of a small cherry, 1.5cm long, oval-shaped and a dark blueish or black colour. It's good to try them raw before gathering, to check that you like the flavour. If you are not able to use them soon after gathering, you can freeze them. Add them to muffins or brownies, stew them with honey or sugar and dollop on to cream or porridge, or even incorporate them into a cheesecake.

If your neighbours have fruiting shrubs, ask to sample the berries. You may need to explain what you're doing, in which case you'll very likely be doing them a favour by letting them know they have an unexpected edible in the garden. If you find one you like, ask for the name. If the owner has no idea of the name, never mind! Ask for a cutting and grow it yourself … fuchsias grow well from slips. Refer to a plant directory or scour garden centres to find out what variety it is.

It would be impossible to list every single variety of fuchsia and describe the taste of the berries, so here are two recipes for you to try – one for a sharp berry and one for a sweeter-tasting one – depending on what you discover in your (or a neighbour's) garden.

Sweet Fuchsia Berry Jam

Makes 1 x 300ml jar

200g fuchsia flowers, washed
200g ripe berries
3 medium apples, peeled, cored
  and chopped
3 tablespoons water
200g preserving sugar
juice of 1 lemon

Wash the flowers and berries and remove the stalks. Put the chopped apples into a heavy-bottomed pan with the water. Steam gently with the lid on the pan for about 10 minutes until soft. Add the sugar and lemon juice and stir over a low heat to dissolve the sugar. Add the flowers and berries and bring to a boil, then boil for 10–15 minutes until you reach setting point. Allow to sit for 5 minutes and bottle into warm jars.

Tart (or Peppery)
Fuchsia-Berry Chutney

Makes 2 x 450ml jars

600g apples, peeled, cored and roughly
*   chopped*
200g demerara sugar
1 whole small head of garlic, peeled
*   and sliced lengthways*
450ml vinegar (any kind, but cider
*   vinegar is nice)*
25g salt
25g cayenne pepper or chilli powder
600g shallots, thinly sliced
600g tart or peppery fuchsia berries,
*   washed*

Put the apples, sugar, garlic, vinegar, salt and cayenne pepper into a heavy-bottomed pan. Simmer until soft, but don't let the apples turn into mush; keep it a bit chunky. Take off the heat, cool for 20 minutes, then add the shallots and the fuchsia berries and mix well.

Pack into warm, sterilised jars and, when completely cool, put on the lids.

This chutney will keep for a couple of weeks in a cool, dark place before eating. Once opened, keep refrigerated.

Geraniums and Pelargoniums
Geranium and *Pelargonium*

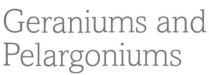

*Flowers range in colour
from whites to dark purples*

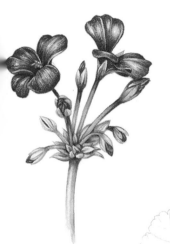

*Pale, fleshy flower stems,
flushed red especially at
opposite end to flower*

*Frilly leaves have circle
of purplish colour, darker
towards centre*

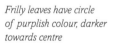

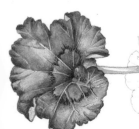

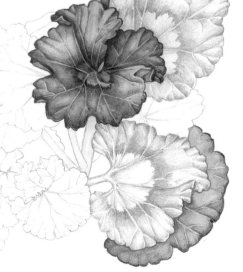

It's no surprise that geraniums and pelargoniums are so popular in our gardens – they are long-lasting plants, which flower continually in the right conditions, care not a hoot for soil types and are propagated easily from either seed or cuttings. Personally, I'm not too keen on the Day-Glo pink ones, but still … there's a lot of variety with this particular plant. And everyone, but everyone, knows exactly what they are! Not everyone knows, however, that the geranium itself (from a Greek word meaning 'crane's bill') is a member of the same family to which pelargonium (meaning 'stork's bill') also belongs. If you're keen to work out which of the two you have on the windowsill, geraniums have five petals of similar size and shape, whereas pelargonium flowers also have five petals but two of the petals are a different size to the other three. Originating in the Mediterranean, these adaptable plants can be found all over the world and there are more than 400 different species for you to choose from. They grow well and prolifically, although they won't survive frost and if they are to survive the winter in colder climates, they will need to be brought indoors before it gets too cold. They prefer being allowed to dry out a little between watering, and regular removal of dead stems will ensure a steady supply of flowers.

Medicinal Use

Geranium oil is used by medical herbalists to reduce anxiety and to help ease the symptoms of PMS and the menopause. It should be avoided during pregnancy. It's also thought that geranium leaf, which has antiseptic properties, can help to heal lesions of the skin, bruises and varicose veins.

Culinary Use

Geraniums and pelargoniums are both edible and the floral leaves and petals of the heavily scented varieties lend a unique flavouring to anything you care to add them to. Flavours range from lemony (*P. crispum*) to rose (*P. graveolens*) to nutmeg (*P. fragrans*) and even cinnamon, coconut, strawberry, pineapple and orange … although some have a rather unpleasant smell and are best avoided, in the kitchen at least. And you don't need to know the full Latin species name to buy the flavour you want. The easiest way to transfer the flavour of the leaves to your baking is simply to line the bottom of your baking tin with the leaves, as in the recipe opposite.

Geranium Sugar

Makes 500g

Take a clean, dry 500ml jar and into it tip 500g caster sugar along with half a dozen clean, dry geranium leaves, buried in the sugar. The scent of the leaves will suffuse the sugar in a matter of just a few days. If you're thinking ahead, you could use some of that sugar to give the following delicious cake an even more powerful geranium aroma.

Rose-Geranium Angel Cake

You can also use lemon rose-geraniums in this recipe, if you have them.

Serves 6–8

6 rose-geranium leaves, washed
250g self-raising flour
a pinch of baking powder
300g golden caster sugar or
    geranium sugar (see recipe left)
12 egg whites
1 teaspoon vanilla extract
2 teaspoons cream of tartar
a pinch of salt

To garnish
rose-geranium flower heads
fresh berries
crème fraiche

Preheat the oven to 200°C/gas 6. Grease a 20cm cake tin and line with parchment paper. Arrange the geranium leaves in the bottom of the tin.

Sift the flour and baking powder together in a bowl and add about 225g of the sugar.

Put the egg whites, vanilla, cream of tartar and salt in a separate, large, clean bowl (the cream of tartar stops the egg whites from separating) and whisk to the soft-peak stage (where the whites are firm but still 'wet'). Using a metal spoon, gently fold in the flour mixture a little at a time, keeping the mixture as airy as possible.

Pour the batter on top of the geranium leaves in the baking tin and bake for about 50 minutes, or until the top of the cake is golden and is springy to the touch.

Remove the cake from the oven, sprinkle the remaining sugar on top whilst still hot and leave in its tin to cool completely. When the cake has cooled, run a palette knife around the edges of the tin and turn the cake out on to a serving plate.

Serve garnished with fresh geranium flowers, berries and crème fraiche.

Geranium Tea

You can make an infusion with the fresh leaves, but drying them first will give a stronger flavour. Simply line a baking tray with parchment paper and spread the leaves on the tray. Leave in a warm, dry place until the leaves are completely dry. Store in an airtight jar until needed – they will keep indefinitely.

To make the tea, simply cover a teaspoon of the leaves with boiling water and steep for about 10 minutes. Add sugar or honey if you wish.

Geranium Syrup

Makes approx. 1 litre

250g golden caster sugar
1 litre boiling water
10–15 fresh geranium leaves (amount
    depends on the size of the leaf)

Put the sugar in a large, heatproof bowl and pour the boiling water over it. Stir until the sugar has dissolved.

Leave the syrup to cool completely, then add the geranium leaves. Leave for up to 6 hours, tasting the syrup at regular intervals. When the syrup has taken the flavour you desire, remove the leaves. Store, frozen, in bottles, remembering to leave a few centimetres at the top of the bottle to allow for expansion.

The syrup is delicious drizzled over cakes, ice-creams and sorbets or poured over waffles and served with a dollop of fresh cream.

Poached Peaches in Geranium-Wine Syrup

Serves 4

4 large very ripe peaches
zest and juice of 1 large unwaxed
    lemon
8 scented geranium leaves
8 tablespoons geranium sugar
    (see page 95)
200ml white wine
whipped cream, to serve

Peel the peaches, leaving as much of the flesh intact as possible, cut in half and remove the stones. Put the peaches, flat-side down, in one layer in a large non-reactive pan (with a lid). Pour half the lemon juice over the peaches and sprinkle with the lemon zest. Scatter the geranium leaves and sugar over them. Cover and cook over a medium heat for about 4 minutes; the juices from the peaches will start to bubble.

Remove from the heat and turn the peaches, add the wine and the rest of the lemon juice, give the pan a shake, then cover and cook for a further 4 minutes.

Using a slotted spoon, carefully transfer the peaches to a serving dish. Remove and discard the geranium leaves and pour the wine and juices from the pan over the peaches. Serve with whipped cream.

Hazel

Corylus avellana

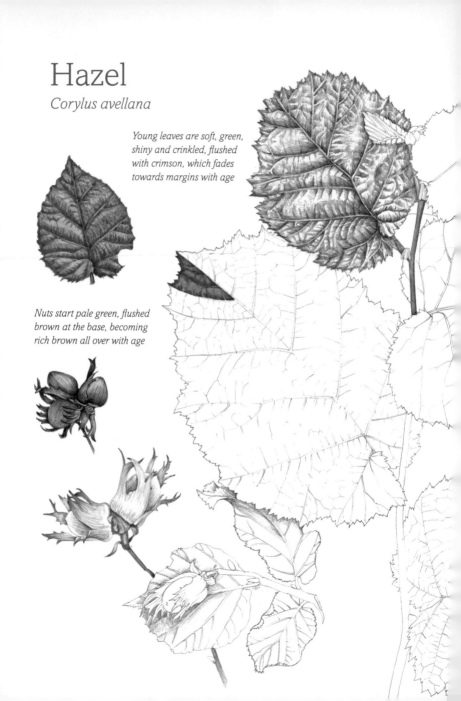

Young leaves are soft, green, shiny and crinkled, flushed with crimson, which fades towards margins with age

Nuts start pale green, flushed brown at the base, becoming rich brown all over with age

Hazel comes from the Anglo-Saxon word *haesel*, meaning 'hat'; hence *haesel knut*, a nut wearing a hat. Which, when you think about it, is very appropriate.

Although hazel grows as a wild hedgerow plant, it is often found in gardens too, as it is such a neat and attractive tree. Personally, I think every garden, large or small, should try to squeeze in one hazel tree at the very least since they're so pretty as well as useful. If you're planting a boundary hedge, hazel is a perfect choice, too. There's also a very unusual twisted hazel (*Corylus avellana* 'Contorta'), which is often used as an ornamental for its spiralling stems and branches. This is not the variety to plant, however, if nuts are your aim. I find that children are very keen on tending and nurturing a young hazel tree once they realise that their favourite 'chocolate' spread is in fact composed primarily of hazelnuts! (see recipe for hazelnut chocolate spread, page 101).

The hazelnut figures prominently in Celtic folklore and is considered a sacred food. Where food was scarce, any source of wild food that provided such good nutrition would have been riches indeed. In addition, hazel trees often grow in clusters of three, a magic number. Bundles of nine hazelnuts are considered to be extraordinarily lucky. Nuts in general were also considered to be a symbol of fertility – hence 'nuts' as a slang term for male genitalia. Yes, really! For some, the hazelnut symbolised wisdom, too, and folklore tells us that if you woo your loved one underneath a hazel tree then, apparently, you're guaranteed to get lucky. And if you were to find a double hazelnut, then you might want to keep it in your pocket to ward off toothache. The efficacy of this method is untested, though, and I suspect that any decent dentist would advise against using this method instead of going for your routine check-up.

Hazels grow all over the planet, from the Americas, throughout Europe and Asia and into Tibet and the Himalayas. Some people call hazelnuts 'filberts' but the two are slightly different. *Corylus maxima* is the filbert proper, but both are called cobnuts. The two plants often hybridise. All varieties of hazelnuts are delicious to eat. Filberts get their name from St Philbert's Day, the 22nd of August, which is the day when the nuts are generally ripe and ready to eat. A hazelnut tree left to grow will reach a height of 6m and about the same in width, but they can be kept in check by careful pruning and even coppicing. The deciduous leaves are a soft green, a little like beech leaves or hornbeam, with serrations. Happy in semi-shade but more likely to produce nuts in a sunnier spot, the hazel takes only two to three years before it fruits. All you need to do after that is find a way of beating the squirrels to the nuts; annoyingly, they will pluck the early nuts, bite out a chunk, find they're unripe and throw them away. However, almost-ripe nuts will mature happily off the tree, laid on newspaper indoors, away from squirrels or peckish family members.

Common Names and Species
Cobnuts, *C. americana*, *C. maxima*.

Medicinal Use
Native Americans used hazel bark as an infusion to soothe high temperatures, although this practice has largely fallen out of use. Hazelnuts are the perfect snack: they contain many minerals and trace elements including iron, magnesium and zinc, as well as niacin and thiamine and polyunsaturated fats, which help protect the heart.

Culinary Use
Many recipes call for hazelnuts to be blanched to remove the skins. Simply pour boiling water over the nuts, leave for 5 minutes, then put them in a sieve and run cold water over them. The skins will come away easily.

Hazelnut Nougat

Makes 25–30 sweets

250g hazelnuts, blanched
1 large egg white
250g white granulated sugar
125g runny honey
250g liquid glucose
3–4 tablespoons water

Line a 22 x 32cm baking tray with rice paper and spread out the hazelnuts in the tray.

Beat the egg white in a squeaky-clean metal bowl until it forms stiff peaks.

Put the sugar, honey, glucose and water in a heavy-bottomed pan and bring to the boil over a low heat initially, stirring to prevent burning. Cook until thick or, if you have a sugar thermometer, to 137°C, then immediately remove the pan from the heat. Gradually whisk the mixture into the egg white. Continue to whisk vigorously for a couple of minutes, or until the mixture turns white and stiffens – it will become difficult to whisk, but carry on until you can't whisk any more – then spoon over the nuts in the prepared tray. Leave for a couple of hours to harden. Crack or chop the nougat into bite-sized pieces.

Hazelnut Chocolate Spread

Children will LOVE making this! If you like, try using white chocolate for a twist.

Makes 500ml

100g hazelnuts, blanched
450g milk chocolate, broken into pieces
75g cocoa powder, sifted
125ml vegetable oil
½ teaspoon vanilla extract

Preheat the oven to 190°C/gas 5. Line a baking tray with parchment paper.

Spread out the nuts on the prepared baking tray, place in the oven and toast until golden, shaking them occasionally and making sure that they don't scorch. Set aside to cool.

Melt the chocolate in a heatproof bowl over a pan of simmering water, making sure that the bowl doesn't touch the water. Set aside to cool.

Put the toasted hazelnuts in a food processor and chop finely. Add the cocoa powder and whizz for a few more seconds. Then add the melted chocolate, the oil and vanilla and whizz again until you have the desired texture. With a spatula, scoop the spread into a warm, sterilised, wide-mouthed jar and, when cool, put on the lid. You'll have plenty of volunteers to help you clear away any leftovers.

Spread over toast or crumpets or, even better, add a warmed-up tablespoonful to the blender when making a banana milkshake.

Hibiscus

Hibiscus

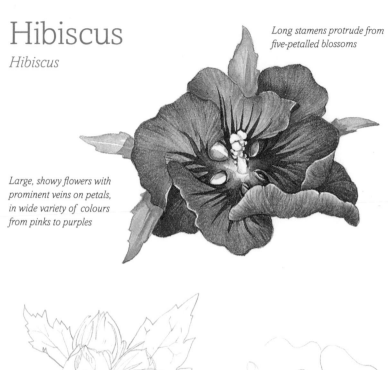

Long stamens protrude from
five-petalled blossoms

Large, showy flowers with
prominent veins on petals,
in wide variety of colours
from pinks to purples

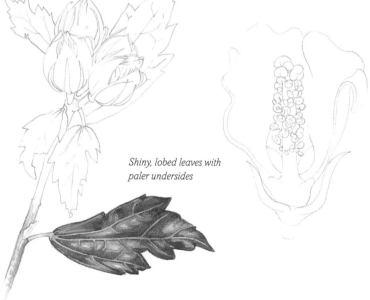

Shiny, lobed leaves with
paler undersides

This lovely flower belongs to the same family as the mallow (see page 152). The name hibiscus comes from the Greek word *iviscos*, meaning 'viscous' or 'sticky'. If you squeeze the stems or petals, you do indeed end up with sticky fingers from the mucilage in the plant.

Hibiscus flowers are large, showy blossoms with a rather sexy bunch of long stamens, which, in many species, protrude from the centre of the five-petalled blossoms. The flowers come in lots of colours and the plant ranges in size from a small shrub to a large tree. Left to its own devices, a hibiscus will grow to the height of a small rowan tree – about 4m – although in gardens they're often trained into standard shapes. The leaves are shaped a bit like oak leaves.

Originating in tropical, subtropical and temperate climates, the hibiscus likes a warm, damp atmosphere, but will happily grow in cooler places too, while a rich, fertilised soil and an open, sunny aspect helps the plant produce those lovely flowers. They also thrive in the Middle East, which is known for its cold nights and chilly winters. Despite its exotic origins, the hibiscus is very widely available and even sold in supermarkets as a pot plant.

The hibiscus flower is believed to be the favourite of the Hindu goddess Kali, so she is often depicted with it; you might also notice fresh blossoms placed by statues of the goddess. And when Gauguin painted his Tahitian beauties with a single hibiscus flower tucked into their hair, did he realise that this was a sign of a single girl?

Common Names and Species

Also known as China rose (*H. rosa-sinensis*), cranberry hibiscus and African rosemallow (*H. acetosella*) or red sorrel (*H. sabdariffa*), *H. syriacus* is illustrated opposite.

Medicinal Use

Research carried out by the American Heart Association has found that hibiscus tea helps to lower blood pressure. You can buy several types of commercial hibiscus-based remedies in health-food stores. Otherwise, people who suffer from kidney problems use the tea as a mild diuretic. In Ayurvedic medicine, hibiscus is used, among other things, to reduce hair loss. Hibiscus is thought to strengthen hair and promote healthy hair growth: hibiscus leaves and flowers, crushed with a little water or a few drops of olive oil, form a lathery paste and can be used as a shampoo.

Culinary Use

Depending on the variety of hibiscus, different parts of the plant are edible. Both the flowers and the leaves of

H. rosa-sinensis (China rose) and *H. sabdariffa* (red sorrel, which you might also find labelled 'roselle') are used for tea. The flowers produce a sweeter flavour and the leaves taste more astringent – try the two together. If you're on holiday in Egypt you might be handed a glass of *karkadé*, Egyptian hibiscus tea. The flowers taste like a cross between rosehips and rhubarb; drying the petals definitely intensifies the flavour. The soft young leaves at the beginning of the season can be cooked like any other green vegetable, steamed and served with butter and a little lemon juice. They have a slight tang of lemon, as do the stalks.

The cranberry hibiscus (*H. acetosella*) tastes rather like cranberries, hence the name. You might see this particular variety described as the African rosemallow.

Hibiscus Tea

This is a popular drink in many parts of the world, known as *karkadé* in Egypt, *bissap* in West Africa, *agua de Jamaica* in Mexico, and *gudhal* in India.

You will need (in volume) one part dried hibiscus petals – either dry your own or buy them – to three parts water and two parts sugar.

Simply soak the petals in the water for about 3 hours, then bring them to the boil. Strain, set the liquid to one side and repeat the process with the same amount of water until the petals have faded in colour. Put all the 'juice' together and add the sugar, stirring to dissolve.

Hibiscus Syrup

Ridiculously simple and totally delicious, hibiscus syrup is a great way to start experimenting with this lovely ingredient. You can use fresh or dried flowers but dried will give a stronger flavour.

Makes 250ml

5g fresh or dried hibiscus flowers
  (dried will give a stronger flavour)
250ml water
100g golden caster sugar

Put the hibiscus flowers and water in a non-reactive pan and bring to the boil. As soon as it comes to the boil, remove from the heat and cover the pan. Set aside to infuse for at least 30 minutes, then strain through a fine-meshed sieve. The water will be a lovely ruby colour.

Return the strained liquid to the pan, add the sugar and stir over a low heat until dissolved. Turn up the heat and cook for 20–30 minutes, or until the mixture has thickened to a syrup. Leave to cool completely and then transfer to a sterilised bottle.

The syrup can be added to prosecco or champagne, drizzled over ice-cream or porridge, stirred into yoghurt or crème fraiche or diluted and drunk as a cordial. It's also delicious with vodka and lots of ice.

You can also use the syrup in the recipe for the spicy hibiscus chutney, overleaf. Increase the ingredients proportionately to make a larger quantity.

Spicy Hibiscus Chutney

Makes enough to fill 1 x 250ml jar

3 tablespoons sunflower oil
3 small red onions, roughly chopped
1 large cooking apple, peeled and
    roughly chopped
2cm fresh root ginger, grated
1 small fresh red chilli, finely chopped
½ teaspoon salt
4 tablespoons soft dark brown sugar
100ml water
100ml hibiscus syrup (see recipe on
    page 105)
6 tablespoons red wine vinegar
½ teaspoon peppercorns

Heat the oil in a pan, then add the onions and cook gently over a low heat until translucent. Stir frequently and make sure they don't burn. Add the chopped apple and cook for 3 minutes to soften. Add the ginger and chilli, cook for 1 minute, then add the salt, sugar, water and hibiscus syrup. Turn up the heat, and cook, stirring, until the liquid has reduced to about 2 tablespoonfuls. Add the vinegar and reduce again to about 2 tablespoonfuls. Leave to cool slightly, then transfer to a warm, sterilised jar. When it has cooled completely, put the lid on the jar and store in the fridge.

Himalayan Honeysuckle

Leycesteria formosa

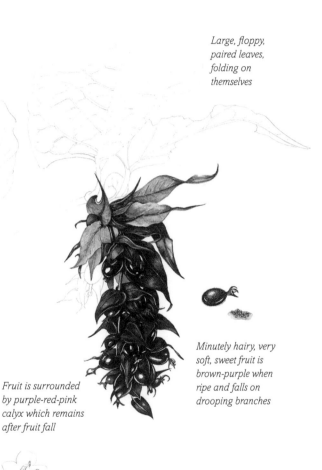

Large, floppy, paired leaves, folding on themselves

Minutely hairy, very soft, sweet fruit is brown-purple when ripe and falls on drooping branches

Fruit is surrounded by purple-red-pink calyx which remains after fruit fall

Although I'd seen this plant many times before, I never knew what it was or that it was edible until I was introduced to it by the head gardener at Victoria Gardens in Neath, South Wales. It was in early October and I collected some of the berries, cooked them and found that the flavour was both unusual and good. I had sent a (rather battered) sample to Lizzie Harper, the illustrator of this book. Luckily, Lizzie spotted some growing in the shrubberies surrounding a school just around the corner from where she lives. I love the fact that our cultivated plants can move ten thousand miles around the planet and still thrive happily in very different climates and conditions.

Himalayan honeysuckle originates in China and the Himalayas. The name is misleading because this plant has no relation at all to the honeysuckle. It's a very graceful and elegant deciduous shrub, a little like a bamboo, growing to some 2m high and wide, and it thrives if cut right back in the early spring. Its new shoots are a blue-green colour and the leaves are narrow, dark green ovals. Although Himalayan honeysuckle is deciduous, the leaves will survive the winter in mild areas. The flowers start to bloom in late summer to early autumn, and these are what make the plant rather special. Small, funnel-shaped blossoms, a little like bell heather, appear at the ends of a series of dangling reddish-purple bracts whose leaves curve gracefully upwards. The whole effect is that of a shrub covered in upside-down mini pagodas. The little flowers at the ends of the bracts are followed by brownish-mauve berries which are well worth harvesting. They have a caramelly chocolate flavour, albeit with an interesting, slightly scorched taste.

Himalayan honeysuckle had its heyday during the Victorian era, but it seems to be making a comeback. It likes fertile, well-drained soil and sunny conditions, but evidently, if the lush plants in Neath are anything to go by, they don't mind being deluged with rain either, and an established plant will tolerate a fair whack of frost. The plant seeds itself easily or can be propagated by taking softwood cuttings. The hollow stems of this plant can be used for making simple flutes and whistles.

Common Names
Flowering nutmeg, pheasant berry, Himalayan nutmeg, toffee berry.

Culinary Use
The berries of this gorgeous plant ripen at different times, so you might want to freeze them until you have amassed a decent volume. The other disadvantage is that the birds evi-

dently have a taste for chocolatey flavours, so you have to be sharp to beat them to the bush.

The ever-ingenious Fergus the Forager (aka wild-food experimentalist Fergus Drennan) partially dries them and makes a sort of fig roll. They are also great in smoothies.

Frozen Yoghurt with Himalayan-Honeysuckle Ripple

The flavour of the berries is so unusual and this frozen yoghurt ripple sets off the taste beautifully. The advantage of this recipe is that you don't need piles and piles of berries.

Serves 4–6

For the frozen yoghurt
2 large egg yolks
1 large egg
50g golden caster sugar
1 teaspoon vanilla extract
1 teaspoon cornflour
300ml full-fat milk
grated zest of 1 medium unwaxed
    lemon or small orange
250g Greek yoghurt

For the honeysuckle-berry purée
115g honeysuckle berries, washed
30g golden caster sugar
Himalayan-honeysuckle sprigs, for
    decoration

To make the custard for the frozen yoghurt, whisk together the egg yolks, whole egg, sugar, vanilla and cornflour in a large bowl until creamy.

In a heavy-bottomed pan, gently heat the milk with the zest and, just before it comes to the boil, remove from the heat and pour over the egg mixture, stirring vigorously. Pour the custard back into the pan and cook over a low heat, stirring, until it starts to thicken. Set aside to cool.

When the custard is completely cool, add the yoghurt and beat with a wooden spoon to combine well. Then either pour into an ice-cream maker and follow the manufacturer's instructions, or pour the mixture into a suitable container and freeze for 2 hours.

To make the purée, put the berries, sugar and a little water in a pan and use a wooden spoon to mash the berries and release their juice. Heat gently until the sugar has dissolved, then remove from the heat. Pass the mixture through a fine-meshed sieve to make a smooth purée.

Remove the container from the freezer, and vigorously stir the frozen yoghurt with a fork and whisk to break up any ice crystals and give a smooth texture. Swirl the purée into the frozen yoghurt, then return to the freezer overnight. Decorate each serving with a sprig of the plant.

Himalayan-Honeysuckle Berry and Apple Cake (with Caramel Topping)

Serves 6–8

For the sponge
450g cooking apples, peeled, cored and chopped
150g Himalayan-honeysuckle berries, washed
115g self-raising flour
1 teaspoon baking powder
115g golden caster sugar
90ml whole milk
50g butter, melted
2 medium eggs

For the topping
75g butter, softened
115g golden caster sugar
1 medium egg
icing sugar, sifted, for dusting

Preheat the oven to 160°C/gas 3. Grease and line a 23cm sandwich tin.

To make the sponge, put the chopped apples and the berries in the bottom of the tin, covering the base. Put the remaining sponge ingredients into a bowl and beat until smooth. Pour the cake mix on top of the apples and berries in the tin, level the top with a spatula and bake for 45 minutes until a light golden colour.

While the cake is baking, cream together the topping ingredients (except for the icing sugar) with the egg. Remove the cake from the oven and spoon the topping over it.

Return the cake to the oven and bake for a further 25 minutes until golden brown and smelling of caramel. Let the cake cool completely in the tin before turning out. Dust with the icing sugar and serve with a dollop of whipped cream.

Hops
Humulus lupulus

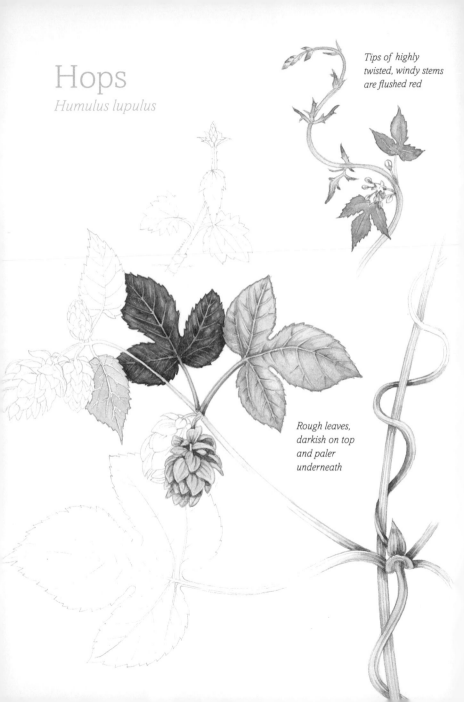

Tips of highly twisted, windy stems are flushed red

Rough leaves, darkish on top and paler underneath

A curious name, this. It was called 'little wolf', according to Pliny, because, he said, it 'strangles' other plants and supports by its 'light, climbing embraces, as the wolf does a sheep'. This last bit sounds tenuous to me. 'Hop' is from an Anglo-Saxon term *hoppan*, meaning 'to climb', and refers, strictly speaking, to the flower. The leaves of this plant are heart-shaped, darkening with age from a pale pistachio green to a darker hue.

Hops grow both in cultivated gardens, where they are generally to be found climbing up trellises, and in the wild, where their small, delicate, paper-textured flowers appear in late summer and early autumn, tumbling up, over and across hedgerows. The flowers look more like a sort of insect carapace than a blossom. It's the flavour of hops that gives beer its distinctive bitterness. Before we used hops for this purpose, that bitter flavour was derived from other plants such as yarrow, broom or even ground ivy. The use of the plant by the Vikings in making beer is reflected in the word 'ale', which is derived from the Viking word for the plant, *öl*.

Hops have been used in Dutch and German beers since the tenth century. However, all parts of the plant are edible. There's even a commercial hop candy (albeit a by-product of brewing) available in the US called B-Hoppy!

The hop, the county flower of Kent, actually originates in Asia. (Barley, another ingredient of beer, also originates in Asia.) Hops will thrive just about anywhere provided they have moist, deep, nutritious soil, sunshine and some kind of support to scramble upwards. Although the plant looks vine-like, it's actually a bine, the technical term for a plant that climbs by means of its own shoots grasping on to a support; a vine sends out tendrils to do the same job.

Humulus is in the same family as nettles and, like nettles, its tough tendrils can be used to make a fabric. You don't see this fabric very often these days, but at one time, before the First World War, it was common in Sweden.

Common Names
Wolf willow.

Medicinal Use
Hops have long had a reputation for making you drowsy; sleepiness was the common complaint of the hop picker, although this could well have been the effect of a long day outside in the sun since, so far, scientists have failed to discover conclusively any sort of soporific compound in the hops themselves. Despite this, pillows stuffed with hops are said to aid a good night's rest. If you want to try

it for yourself, a hop pillow is very easy to make. Simply fill a small cotton cushion cover or pillowcase with hops, add dried lavender, too, if you have some, and loop over the bedpost. A hop tea – made from the dried leaves, stalks and flowers – is said to be a good liver tonic to drink in spring (if you are considering a detox, this might be worth a try).

Culinary Use

All parts of the hop plant are edible. It was popular with the Romans, who planted it in their gardens as a vegetable. The young shoots – generally prolific – are a delicious vegetable which requires very little preparation; simply cut them close to the ground when they are between 10 and 20cm long, and steam or boil for a few minutes until tender, then drain and serve hot with butter, lemon and pepper. The young, tender leaves, shredded finely, add flavour to a salad. The larger leaves can be used in the same way as vine leaves, to make *dolmades*. The smaller leaves at the ends of the tendrils can also be sautéed. Some older recipes advise soaking the shoots in salted water for a couple of hours to leach away some of the bitter, endive-like flavour.

With hops flowers themselves, a little goes a long way. The flowers are earthy, slightly citric with a weirdly medicinal tang, which may be an acquired taste. They lend themselves very well to using as a rub for sweeter types of meat such as lamb or pork. You can also try infusing them into a custard to make ice-cream or freezing a hop-flower syrup to make an interesting sorbet. Infused into a good olive oil, they add an unusual piquancy to salad dressings or dipping oil.

Serves 4

1 large garlic bulb
400g baby plum tomatoes
6 tablespoons extra-virgin olive oil
2 small ciabatta loaves
petals of 4 fresh hop flowers, picked
    over and washed
a squeeze of lemon
salt and freshly ground pepper, to taste

Preheat the oven to 180°C/gas 4.

Slice off the base of the garlic and wrap the bulb in foil. Slit each of the baby plum tomatoes with a sharp knife and place in a shallow baking tray with a little oil. Place on the top shelf of the oven and roast along with the garlic for about 30 minutes. Stir the tomatoes occasionally so that they roast evenly.

About 10 minutes before the tomatoes and garlic are ready, cut each ciabatta in half lengthways and brush with oil. Scorch the bread on a griddle, cover with foil and place on the bottom rack of the oven to keep warm.

Remove the tomatoes and garlic from the oven. Put the tomatoes in a bowl. Remove the garlic from the foil and squeeze the flesh from each individual garlic clove into the tomatoes. Add a glug of olive oil, the fresh hop petals, lemon juice and salt and pepper to taste. Mix well.

Remove the ciabatta halves from the oven and top each half with the tomato mix. Serve with a green salad.

Makes 2 x 450ml jars

120g hop shoots, washed
120ml water
120g spring onions
1 large red pepper
30g sundried tomatoes (in oil)
120g cucumber
1 red onion
30g capers
I teaspoon finely chopped fresh parsley
a few drops of balsamic vinegar
salt and freshly ground black pepper,
    to taste
100ml olive oil

First, steam the hop shoots for about 5 minutes in the water or until tender. Leave to cool. Chop the cooled hop shoots and all the other vegetables to roughly the same size and put in a large bowl. Add all the other ingredients (except for the oil), season well and, finally, pour in the oil. Mix everything together well and set aside to marinate for about 1 hour.

Serve as a side dish alongside cold meats and cheeses, or on top of toast, or add to a salad. The relish is best eaten right away, but will keep, covered, in the fridge for a day or two.

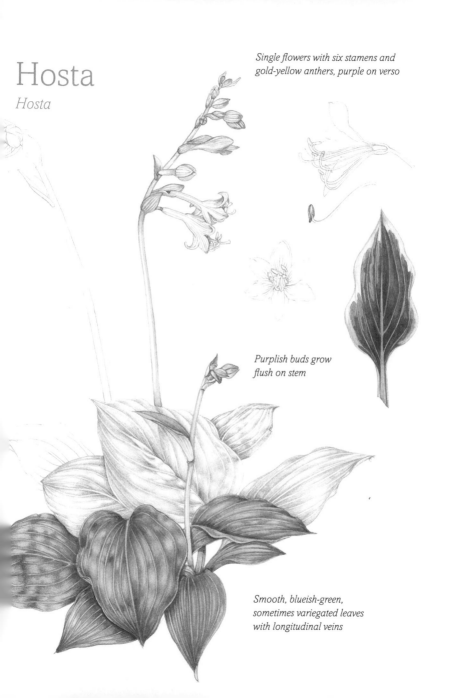

Hosta
Hosta

Single flowers with six stamens and
gold-yellow anthers, purple on verso

Purplish buds grow
flush on stem

Smooth, blueish-green,
sometimes variegated leaves
with longitudinal veins

Native to north-east Asia (specifically China), hostas were named after the explorer who first discovered them, Nicolaus Host. They are sometimes referred to as plantain lilies or funkia (a term largely obsolete these days, after the German botanist Heinrich Christian Funck). Hostas are generally grown for their highly decorative foliage: lavish, abundant clumps of smooth, floppy, spear-shaped leaves in different shades of green. They are shade-tolerant, hardy and easily propagated, but what makes generally peaceable hosta enthusiasts gnash their teeth and turn their thoughts towards violence are slugs and snails, which will devour them in a flash if given the opportunity, so the best way to protect hostas is to grow them in pots. Alternatively, to keep slugs away from your hostas without resorting to chemical weapons, pull off some leaves from the outer edges of the plants and encircle the plants with them – the slugs will congregate under this barrier of leaves. Then you can simply remove the slugs into a bucket and put them somewhere else – and hopefully keep your hostas intact.

Hostas are delicious, and not just to slugs and snails. In Japan the plant is known as *giboshi* and sold as a vegetable, *urui*. There, as in China, hostas grow as abundantly as weeds, bordering the paddy fields. Hostas, specifically the *sieboldiana* variety, are an important cash crop in the mountain villages of Hokkaido in Japan. *H. sieboldiana* and *H. montana* tend to be recommended for culinary uses, but it's worth experimenting with whatever you have to hand.

Common Names
Plantain lily, funkia, giboshi.

Medicinal Use
Chinese herbal medicine used hosta flowers in treatments for cancer; however, there is no scientific evidence yet that the treatment is effective or otherwise.

Culinary Use
All of the hosta is edible – leaves, flowers and shoots. The taste is a bit like spinach, cos lettuce or pea shoots. And the beauty of hostas is that, so long as you can hold the slugs at bay, they have a long growing season, even in colder climates, and the plants don't mind being chopped back to ground level – a real 'cut and come again' crop. The gardens at Highgrove are home to a huge collection of the larger-leaved varieties and one wonders if Prince Charles is aware of the versatility of these plants in the kitchen. The leaves and shoots can be used in stir-fries like spinach, as a general pot herb, or steamed with lemon juice and butter

in the same way as asparagus. You can also make *hostakopita* (the Greek feta-and-filo pie), using hosta leaves for the filling. To harvest the leaves for cooking, use kitchen scissors or a sharp knife and cut them as close to the ground as possible, leaving the crown to continue to grow.

Urui with Honey Mustard Dressing

Serves 4 as a side dish

20 fresh hosta leaves
a pinch of salt
1 tablespoon toasted sesame seeds

For the dressing
2 tablespoons olive oil
1 tablespoon runny honey
½ tablespoon wholegrain mustard
2 teaspoons balsamic vinegar
1 teaspoon soy sauce
salt and freshly ground black pepper,
*   to taste*

First, make the dressing. Put all the ingredients in a bowl and whisk vigorously. Alternatively, put all the ingredients in a jar, put on the lid and shake vigorously to combine.

Wash the hosta leaves well and cook in a pan of boiling water with a pinch of salt for 1½ minutes. Drain the leaves and cut into 2cm slices. Toss the leaves in the dressing, scatter the sesame seeds over the top and serve immediately.

Japanese Quince
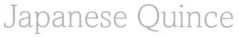
Chaenomeles japonica

*Rough, matt leaves with
tiny serrated margins*

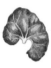

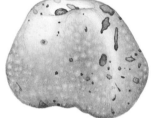

*Fruits are very hard
and very fragrant*

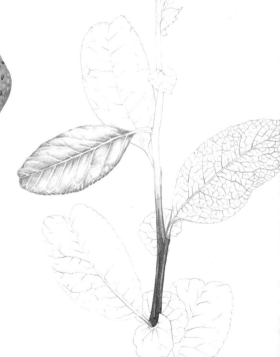

Although they are related, the ornamental quinces – *Chaenomeles* – are distinctly different from the real quince, *Cydonia oblonga*, a tree that, sadly, is not often seen these days. Although ornamental quinces originated in Asia, they are popular garden plants and their hard fruits, borne on spiky branches from late summer onwards, are fragrantly tasty and generally abundant.

Probably the most popular is the Japanese ornamental quince, *C. japonica*, whose small flowers are a cheery reddish-orange. All ornamental quinces have edible fruits, but if you've tried to bite into one of the raw fruits you'd very likely be put off as they're incredibly hard. Cooked, however, it's a different story.

Medicinal Use

In Japan, the use of this quince as a medicine is mentioned in records written at least 300 years ago. Its use as an effective cough medicine in ancient times is backed up by recent testing – it has anti-inflammatory, anti-bacterial properties and so is soothing for sore throats. Another benefit is that there is more vitamin C in a Japanese quince than in a lemon.

Culinary Use

Although we tend to associate marmalade with oranges (particularly those bitter ones from Seville) the original 'marmalade' was a preserve made from quinces. The word marmalade actually comes from the Portuguese word for the quince, *marmelo*. Quinces are very high in pectin and so will set very easily, lending themselves well to jam and jelly making.

Membrillo

This is the Spanish word not only for the quince plant and fruit but also for the delicious thick paste made from the fruit, which is traditionally served with a chunk of Manchego cheese, itself a delicacy from the Basque region. Although the quince that was originally used for the recipe was the kind that grows on a tree and looks like an apple (*Cydonia oblonga*) the recipe works just as well with the fruits of the ornamental quince. With thanks to Louise Gray for the inspiration.

Makes 4 x 450g jars

2kg Japanese quinces, washed, depipped, cored and chopped
1 whole vanilla pod
juice and zest of 1 unwaxed lemon
white caster sugar (see method for amount)

Line a 20 x 20cm baking tray with greaseproof paper.

Put the chopped quince, vanilla pod and the lemon juice and zest into a heavy-bottomed pan and just cover with water. Cover and cook on a low heat for about 1 hour or until the fruit is soft. The kitchen will fill up with a delightful fragrance, a cross between apples and pears.

Remove the vanilla pod, drain the cooked fruit pulp and weigh it. Then weigh out the same amount of sugar.

Remove any pips remaining in the pulp, then, using a stick blender, blend the fruit until it is silky smooth. Return the pulp to the pan, add the equivalent weight of sugar and cook, uncovered, on a low heat, stirring, until the sugar has dissolved. Next, cover the pan and cook on a low heat, for a further 60–90 minutes. When the mixture has darkened to a scorched orange colour, remove from the heat, pour into warm jars or into a tray and set aside to cool. Will keep indefinitely in the jars and for a week or so, in the tray, refrigerated.

Jasmine

Jasminum officinale

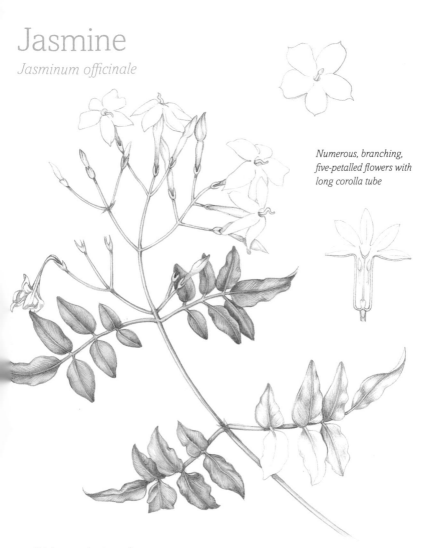

Numerous, branching, five-petalled flowers with long corolla tube

Bright, smooth, pinnate leaves, terminating in sharp apex

The jasmine flower has arguably the most divine scent in the world. This alone is reason enough to grow as much of it as you possibly can. But you can make delicious things to eat with it, too. Not all varieties are edible, however; *J. officinale* and *J. sambac* are the ones to look for if you'd like to grow them for culinary uses. When I lived in London my Greek neighbour had an exuberant jasmine hedge running the length of her garden wall. She used to make long strings of the flowers, running the needle and thread through the centre of each flower and out of the little hole at the back of the blossom, and then hang the scented garlands over the doorways, tacking them up with drawing pins. Her house always smelled amazing.

The jasmine is part of the same family as the olive, *Oleaceae*. It originates in semi-tropical climes in parts of Europe as well as in Asia and Africa, but has made itself at home all over the world, so much so that it was once believed to be indigenous to Switzerland.

An evergreen shrub that goes by the lyrical name of 'moon shine in the garden' in parts of India, a jasmine shrub will grow to about 3m long/high. The plants sold as houseplants in supermarkets can be planted outside, too, and they prefer a good fertile soil and a sunny aspect. Jasmine needs a moist, rich, well-drained soil to grow well, plus it needs to be protected from severe frosts or continuous cold temperatures.

J. officinale – the kind grown by my neighbour – forms a large, spreading shrub with a trailing/climbing habit. The flowers are small and white and with a waxy feel and a heavenly scent.

Jasmine is a popular girl's name; it comes from the Persian *yasameen*, meaning 'gift from god', and in Iran *J. officinale* goes by the lovely name of 'poet's jasmine'. In India, women wear jasmine flowers in their hair and they are also woven into *malas*, garlands of fresh flowers presented as offerings to statues and images of deities. In South India you're never far from a jasmine seller, patiently weaving the blossoms into braids.

Common Species
J. sambac, J. officinale.

Medicinal Use
Jasmine oil is used in aromatherapy to lift the spirits, and also as an antidepressant and an aphrodisiac. Inhaling the scent can be both soothing and invigorating and can calm spasms of coughing but, if overused, jasmine oil can cause headaches.

Culinary Use
Although you can make drinks using jasmine, it's not easy to make jasmine

tea at home. Called *mòlĭhu chá* in Chinese, jasmine tea is actually a mixture of green tea or white tea, or sometimes a blend, infused with jasmine flowers of the *sambac* variety to add that distinctive fragrance to the tea leaves through a precise application of temperature and humidity. You can use jasmine tea bags to add flavouring to recipes.

Pick the jasmine on a warm sunny day when the flowers are at their most fragrant, to make the following recipes.

Jasmine Syrup

This fragrant syrup is worth making in large quantities – you can use it to make a delicious jasmine drizzle cake (see overleaf) or you can turn it into a sorbet simply by freezing the syrup and whizzing with a hand blender to a smooth-textured ice.

Makes 2.5 litres

*2 large handfuls of fresh
    jasmine flowers
1kg golden caster sugar
2 litres boiling water*

Pick over and wash the jasmine flowers.

Put the sugar in a large non-reactive (glass or stainless-steel) jug or bowl and pour the boiling water on top. Stir until the sugar is dissolved, then leave to cool.

Once it has cooled, throw in the flowers, stir and set aside to infuse for up to 6 hours. Test and when you are happy with the flavour, strain into a jug and then pour into sterilised bottles or jars. (You can store in clean plastic water bottles and freeze, but be sure to leave a few centimetres of room in the bottle to allow for expansion when frozen.)

Jasmine Drizzle Cake

Serves 6–8

225g butter, at room temperature, plus
*   extra for greasing*
225g golden caster sugar
zest of 1 unwaxed lime
4 large eggs, beaten
225g self-raising flour
2 tablespoons hot water, as needed
150ml jasmine syrup (see recipe on
*   page 125)*
2–3 tablespoons white granulated sugar

Preheat the oven to 180°C/gas 4. Grease a deep 20cm round baking tin, preferably a springform tin, and line with parchment paper.

In a mixing bowl, cream the butter, caster sugar and lime zest until pale and fluffy. Add the beaten egg a little at a time, whisking well after each addition until thoroughly combined. Sift in 1 tablespoon of the flour with the last addition of egg, then sift in the remaining flour and fold it in gently (adding the hot water if necessary) with a metal spoon until thoroughly combined. Spoon the mixture into the baking tin, level the top with a spatula and bake for 45 minutes or until an inserted skewer comes out clean.

Remove from the oven and leave the cake to cool in its tin for 5 minutes, then insert the skewer all the way through the cake at regular, 2cm intervals. Pour the jasmine syrup evenly over the cake – don't worry if some of it sits at the edges, as it will all soak in. Sprinkle the granulated sugar over the top and return to the oven for 5 minutes. Remove from the oven and leave to cool completely before turning the cake out on to a serving plate.

Jasmine and Rose Lemonade

Serves 8

25 jasmine flowers
10 fresh, strongly scented rose petals
5 tablespoons white caster sugar
500ml boiling water
500ml ice-cold water
juice of 1 large lemon

Pick over and wash the flowers and petals.

Put the sugar in a heatproof jug or bowl, pour the boiling water over it and stir until the sugar has dissolved. Add the cold water and leave to cool to room temperature. Add the jasmine flowers, rose petals and lemon juice and leave to steep for 8 hours, or overnight. Serve over ice in tall glasses.

Juneberry

Amelanchier

*Showy red fruit pomes become dark
purple, bluish-black when ripe*

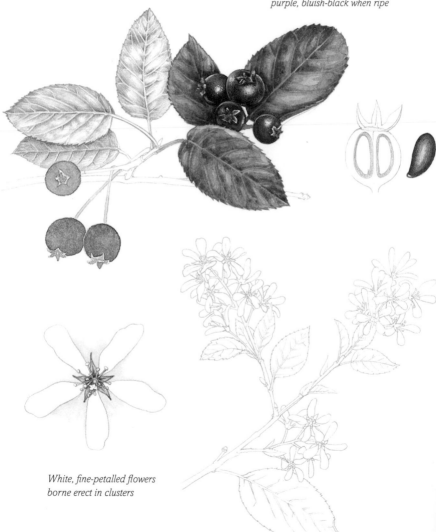

*White, fine-petalled flowers
borne erect in clusters*

At one time, in the Appalachian mountains of New England, the appearance of the little white blossoms on the juneberry tree in the springtime was a sign that the ground had defrosted enough to bury those who had died during the winter months; hence one possible explanation for the name 'service tree', for the funeral ceremonies that would follow. A more prosaic (and possibly tenuous) explanation is that the tree looks rather like a rowan, whose Latin name, *Sorbus*, sounds a bit like 'service'. This change in the season from winter to spring also heralded the time that the river herrings – also known as shads – would start to spawn, which explains another name for the tree.

Amelanchier trees belong to the same family as the rose and are native to North America but are also now well-established in the UK and other parts of Europe. There are many different species and varieties of this pretty decidious tree which can grow to 20m tall. The name *Amelanchier*, it is supposed, derives from a corruption of a Gallic word, *amelanco*, meaning 'downy apple'. The largest city of Saskatchewan (Saskatoon) is named after the amelanchier, and the fruits are harvested on a commercial basis under the name of Saskatoon berries. The species that is arguably the most popular in Europe is *A. lamarckii*, a natural hybrid that thrives in just about any conditions, although it doesn't like soggy soil and needs sunshine in order to produce a decent crop of berries. The best-known species in the US are *A. canadensis* (originating in Canada), illustrated here, and *A. alnifolia*, which gives us the gloriously named Saskatoon berry. All amelanchier berries are edible, although the general rule of thumb is that the darker the berry, the juicier and tastier it is. In North America, native peoples such as the Osage and the Omaha used the berries to make pemmican, a very nutritious and infinitely portable foodstuff comprising a highly concentrated blend of dried meats and powdered berries, with a texture not unlike jerky and a similar longevity, made in the same way as fruit leather (that is, by simmering the fruits until they reduce to a thick paste, then spreading the paste thinly on a flat surface and leaving to dry, either in an oven or in the open air).

Common Names and Species
Serviceberry, service tree, shad, shadbush or shadwood, wild pear, chuckley pear, sugarplum, Saskatoon, *A. canadensis*, *A. laevis*, *A. lamarckii*, *A. alnifolia*.

Medicinal Use
The plant isn't used very much

nowadays but the Native Americans had a variety of uses for it, mainly to treat minor ailments such as upset stomachs and to soothe the symptoms of colds. More unusually, a decoction of the bark was used to prevent snow blindness.

Culinary Use

The berries are at their best when fully ripe and purple in colour. Juneberries can be eaten straight from the bush; they are sweet and delicious, with a hint of almond. Given how tasty they are, it's strange that juneberries aren't more widely used here in the UK. The birds love them too, though, so if you have a low-growing shrub you might consider throwing a net over the plant to prevent them taking the choicest fruits.

Cooking with juneberries is easy and there are no pips or seeds to worry about. They also dry well and can be used like currants. Simply spread them on a baking tray and place in a low oven for about 4–5 hours, or in hot, dry weather they can be sundried.

Saskatoon Pie

Serves 6–8

For the pastry
500g plain flour, plus extra for rolling
100g icing sugar
zest of 1 unwaxed orange
200g unsalted butter, plus extra for greasing
a little chilled water

For the filling
800g juneberries, picked over and washed
175g white granulated sugar, plus extra for sprinkling
100ml water
2½ tablespoons ground almonds
zest and juice of 1 unwaxed lemon
1 egg, beaten

Preheat the oven to 220°C/gas 7. Grease a 20cm pie dish.

To make the pastry, sift together the flour and icing sugar into a mixing bowl and stir in the orange zest. Cut the butter into small cubes and rub it into the flour with your fingertips until the mixture resembles fresh breadcrumbs. Mix in the chilled water a little at a time and work lightly to form a soft dough. Put into a plastic bag, or wrap in cling film, and refrigerate.

For the filling, put the berries, sugar and water into a heavy-bottomed pan and simmer for about 10 minutes. Allow to cool a little, then stir in the ground almonds and the lemon zest and juice.

Roll out three-quarters of the chilled pastry on a floured surface to a little larger than the pie dish and line the dish with it. Pour in the filling, then roll out the rest of the pastry so it's large enough to generously cover the pie dish, then cut out a neat 1cm diameter hole in the centre. Carefully lift the pastry over the top of the pie, pressing your thumb into the edges to seal them. Brush the pastry with the beaten egg and sprinkle with the remaining granulated sugar.

Bake for 15 minutes, then reduce the oven temperature to 170°C/gas 3 and bake for a further 30–40 minutes until golden brown.

Serve slightly warm or at room temperature with cream or ice-cream.

Juneberry Jelly

Makes enough to fill 3 x 450g jars

1kg (or more) ripe purple juneberries
250g preserving sugar (with added
*   pectin) per 250ml juice (see method)*
pectin powder

Pick over the berries and remove the stalks. Wash the berries, put them into a heavy-bottomed pan and use a potato masher or wooden spoon to lightly mash them. Add water to cover and simmer on a low heat for about 15 minutes.

Strain the fruit mixture through a jelly bag into a large bowl; squeeze the bag if you don't mind a cloudy jelly, or drain overnight for a clear, jewel-like jelly.

Measure the strained juice and weigh out the sugar – 250g per 250ml juice.

Return the juice to the pan along with the sugar and heat until the sugar has dissolved. Clip a sugar thermometer to the inside of the pan, if you have one. Turn up the heat and bring the juice to the boil. Remove any foam with a slotted spoon and boil the mixture until it reaches 104°C, or use the cold saucer method (see page 13) to see if it has reached setting point. Pour the jelly into warm, sterilised jars and seal with waxed discs. When the jelly is cold, put on the lids.

Juneberry Garibaldi Biscuits

Makes 12–15 biscuits, depending on their size

90g white caster sugar, plus 60g for sprinkling
90g cold butter, diced, plus extra for greasing
380g self-raising flour, plus extra for rolling
a pinch of salt
250g dried juneberries, finely chopped
90ml whole milk
3–4 tablespoons cold water
1 egg white, beaten

Preheat the oven to 190°C/gas 5. Grease a large baking tray and line with parchment paper.

In a bowl, cream 90g of the sugar with the butter until pale and fluffy. Sift in the flour and salt and beat until combined. Stir in 80g of the chopped dried juneberries and gradually stir in the milk. Knead the mixture lightly until combined and a soft dough forms. Wrap the dough in cling film and refrigerate for 30 minutes.

Put the remaining juneberries in a food processor with 3–4 tablespoons of water and blend to a paste.

Remove the dough from the fridge, cut in half and roll each half out on a floured board to a thickness of 1cm. Spread the fruit paste evenly over one of the sheets of dough, place the other sheet of dough on top and, very carefully, roll again to a thickness of 4–5mm. Cover with cling film and refrigerate on the board for 30 minutes.

Remove the dough from the fridge, brush with the egg white and sprinkle with the rest of the sugar. Cut the dough into 12–15 rectangles, each measuring about 12 x 15cm, then place on the prepared baking tray, leaving enough space between each one to allow them to spread. Bake for 8 minutes, turning the tray halfway through the cooking time. Leave to cool.

Juniper

Juniperus communis

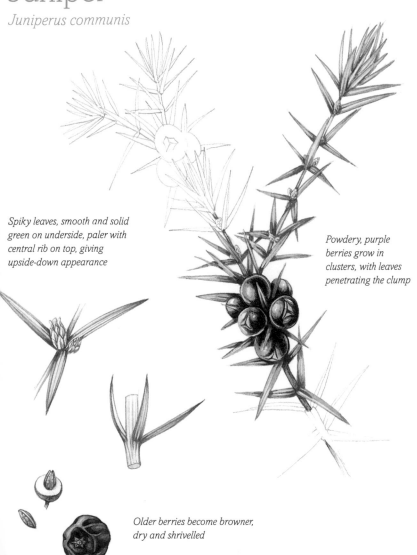

Spiky leaves, smooth and solid green on underside, paler with central rib on top, giving upside-down appearance

Powdery, purple berries grow in clusters, with leaves penetrating the clump

Older berries become browner, dry and shrivelled

There are at least 50 species of juniper, which is a part of the cypress (*Cupressaceae*) family. It's difficult to pinpoint a specific country of origin, but the juniper is found widely throughout the northern hemisphere. Junipers are grown in many gardens, yet it's safe to say many owners won't realise that this evergreen is the source of the juniper berry, commonly used to flavour gin. Gin was invented by a Dutch doctor, Franciscus Sylvius, as a medicine designed to have a diuretic effect. In the 17th century this highly alcoholic 'tonic' was incredibly cheap and resulted in a generation of alcoholics, including children. Thankfully, those days are gone, and gins today have become ever more sophisticated and are flavoured with various botanicals. To make gin, the juniper berries are used while they are still green and they are also an ingredient in the liqueur chartreuse.

Juniper berries are not actually berries but modified cones, which take between 6 and 18 months to reach maturity. The berries of the common juniper (*J. communis*) are the most widely used, but not all juniper berries are edible and those of the *J. sabina* species are in fact poisonous. If you're planning on planting a juniper, you can choose from a variety of different styles, colours and shapes. Some will grow to narrow trees as high as 40m, while others are low-growing shrubs.

The berries of the common juniper start out green, maturing to a dark purple. Each berry has a seed inside and is too bitter to be eaten directly from the tree.

Common Species
J. drupacea, J. phoenicea, J. californica.

Medicinal Use
Juniper berries can cause uterine contractions, resulting in spontaneous abortion, hence the rather grisly, old-fashioned method of terminating a pregnancy with a hot bath and a bottle of gin (a possible reason for gin's nickname, 'mother's ruin'). Therefore juniper products should be avoided during pregnancy. Some Native American tribes have been known to use the berries as a contraceptive and an old American folk remedy used juniper-berry tea as a cure for colds and flu.

Culinary Use
The Romans used juniper berries as a cheaper alternative to black pepper. Today, juniper berries are most used as a spice in Scandinavian cuisine, such as in rich wild game and poultry dishes, as the bitter berries aid digestion. Sauerkraut, the German pickle made from cabbage, is traditionally flavoured with juniper berries.

Juniper-Berry 'Gin'

Gin is made commercially through a process of careful distillation which is beyond the capabilities of most home brewers, but what you can try is this infusion of the berries, which lends an interesting flavour to clear spirits. Use the most neutral gin or vodka and the best quality possible (not a really cheap one). The following recipe is a serious competitor for some of the expensive artisan gins you can buy from specialist spirit-makers; you may also want to experiment with your own mix of herbs, spices, fruits and even flower petals, but start with a few flavourings first and taste before adding more. Unlike the distilled versions, your gin will not be transparent. Rather, it will take on a pretty pink/orange hue from the ingredients used.

Makes 500ml

Note: *You'll need a 1-litre Kilner jar, or similar, in which to infuse the ingredients.*

2 tablespoons fresh or dried juniper
*   berries, washed if fresh*
3 strips of orange zest
500ml good-quality gin or vodka

For the flavourings, choose from:
cardamom pods
cinnamon
mace
fresh coriander seeds
star anise
sweet cicely seeds
fennel seeds
lemongrass
liquorice root

Put the juniper berries and orange zest into the Kilner jar and pour the gin or vodka over them. Seal the jar and leave to infuse at room temperature for 3 days before tasting. You can then experiment with a selection of flavourings (don't use powdered spices or herbs, which will turn to sludge in the bottom of the bottle). Remember to add sweet flavours (star anise, fennel, liquorice root, sweet cicely, etc.) to balance any bitter ones, and don't be tempted to overdo it. The aim is to have a subtly fragranced spirit with sweet and bitter tones.

For example, try a tablespoon each of cardamom pods, fresh coriander seeds and 6 star anise, and leave for a further day before tasting again.

Once you're happy with the taste, simply strain the solids away and decant the flavoured gin or vodka into a clean, sterilised bottle.

Juniper-Berry Jelly

Makes 2 x 300ml jars

500g ripe juniper berries (or 450g dried
* berries, soaked in water overnight)*
150ml apple juice
white granulated sugar (see method for
* amount)*
juice of 1 small lemon

Wash the berries thoroughly. Put them in a pan and just cover with water. Bring to the boil and simmer, half covered, for 1 hour. Remove from the heat, leave to cool, then pour the berries and their cooking water in a food processor and blend to a smooth purée (or use a stick blender). Pass the purée through a fine-meshed sieve into a bowl.

Add the apple juice, then weigh the resulting liquid and add the same quantity of granulated sugar. Put the juice, sugar and lemon juice back into the pan and heat to dissolve the sugar before bringing to a rolling boil. Boil for about 10 minutes and remove any scum that forms on the surface with a slotted spoon. Test for setting point; a sugar thermometer should read 105°C, or you can use the cold saucer test (see page 13). Allow to cool a little before transferring to warm, sterilised jars. When the jelly is completely cold, cover with waxed discs and lid up.

This jelly is a great accompaniment to cold meats or strong cheeses but it can be eaten in sweet dishes too.

Lavender
Lavandula angustifolia

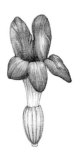

*All parts of plant
are highly scented*

*Calyx flushed purple
towards top margin*

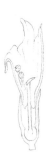

*Fragrant leaves covered
in downy, white hair*

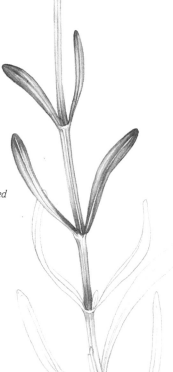

L avender was one of the plants that originally inspired this book: I saw a young plant (most likely treated, however, with all manner of pesticides and chemicals) in a supermarket with the label 'not for human consumption' and it got me thinking. All varieties of lavender are, in fact, fit for human consumption, though admittedly some taste better than others. The best lavenders for edible purposes, luckily, are also the most popular with gardeners and garden centres. These are *Lavandula angustifolia* (*L. officinalis*), 'true lavender', or 'English lavender' (illustrated here), and *Lavandula* x *intermedia*, 'Provence lavender'. If you are not sure which variety of lavender you have or if it is good for cooking, sniff it. If it has a strong medicinal scent, then it will taste that way too. Never use lavender or any other plant as food if you suspect it has been treated with chemicals.

There are many different varieties of lavender, but generally speaking they take the appearance of a shrub, becoming woody with age, with long, slim, greyish leaves and flowers borne at the top of long, skinny stems. The flowers range through a spectrum of blues and purple/blue, which is synonymous with the name of the plant, although some varieties have yellow or even black flowers.

Originating in dry, hot Mediterra-nean territories, lavender is happiest when growing in a dry, sunny climate with well-drained, gravelly soil. Lavender will grow in poor soil conditions and has no need for fertilisers, but very damp conditions are the plant's nemesis, causing its roots to rot.

Common Species and Cultivars
Lavandula atriplicifolia, *L.* x *intermedia*, *L. angustifolia* (also known as *L. officinalis*).

Medicinal Use
A bottle of lavender oil is handy to have in the kitchen, since it really does soothe burns speedily. This was discovered by a French doctor and chemist, René Gattefossé, who accidentally used the oil after burning his hand during a laboratory experiment; the dramatic curative effect of the oil inspired him to investigate further and he discovered that the plant was both antiseptic and analgesic. When you've had a cold, you might have used lavender as the active ingredient in a steam bath to help clear congested nasal passages.

Culinary Use
Few people would enjoy munching on a lavender flower just for the hell of it, but, as a flavouring, it offers unique possibilities. The best way to describe the flavour of the flowers

and the leaves is to tell you that they taste as they smell; a pungent, aromatic, clean and sweetly medicinal flavour, unlike anything else.

Lavender should be used sparingly in the kitchen – too much and the result is an unmistakeable soapy, disinfectant taste. It is no accident that the Romans named the plant *lavandarius*, sharing the same origin as *lavare*, which means 'to wash'.

Use it in place of rosemary – the stems are especially good for this – or use the flowers in a rub for lamb.

Lavender Syrup

Makes 1 litre

Lavender lends itself very well to a syrup; simply measure, in a jug, half a litre of caster sugar and the same amount of water), half a mug of white wine (anything left over in the bottle will be fine) and 2 tablespoons of grape juice. Heat to boiling point, turn down the heat and simmer for 5 minutes. Add 3 tablespoons of chopped fresh lavender flowers, then take the pan off the heat. Allow to stand for 2 hours, then strain the syrup. It's delicious drizzled over strawberries and cream, over Greek yoghurt and toasted almonds, or mixed with sparkling water and poured over ice.

Lavender Lemonade

Serves 4

900ml water
4 tablespoons fresh or dried lavender
   flowers and stalks, washed if fresh
100g white caster sugar
125ml fresh lemon juice

Boil 300ml of the water and steep the flowers and stalks in it for 10–15 minutes. Remove the lavender.

Mix the sugar with the remaining 600ml of water, bring to the boil, then cover and simmer for a couple of minutes. Allow to cool slightly (so you can comfortably put your finger in it), then combine the sugar water, lavender water and lemon juice. Allow to cool before refrigerating. Serve chilled.

Lavender Shortcake Cookies

Makes 20–24 cookies, depending on their size

350g unsalted butter, at room
   temperature, plus extra for greasing
125g golden caster sugar
4 tablespoons icing sugar, sifted
2 tablespoons finely chopped fresh
   lavender flowers
1 tablespoon finely chopped fresh mint
   or basil
finely grated zest of 1 medium unwaxed
   lemon
325g plain flour, sifted, plus extra for
   rolling
65g cornflour
a pinch of table salt

In a bowl, cream together the butter, caster sugar and icing sugar until pale and fluffy. Add the lavender, mint or basil and the lemon zest, and mix until thoroughly combined. Sift together the flour, cornflour and salt into the bowl and beat until the mixture forms a smooth dough. Divide the mixture into two, roll each half into a ball, then wrap each ball separately in cling film and refrigerate for 1 hour.

Preheat the oven to 170°C/gas 3. Grease 2 baking trays and line with parchment paper.

Remove the first ball of dough from the fridge and roll out to 6mm thick on a lightly floured surface. Use a cookie cutter to cut out the biscuits, then place them, spaced out, on the prepared baking trays. Repeat with the remaining dough.

Bake for 15–18 minutes, or until the cookies just turn golden, making sure that they don't overbake. Leave to cool for a few minutes on their trays, then transfer to a wire rack to cool completely.

Lavender and Raspberry Lollies

You can substitute any soft fruit for the raspberries, such as blueberries, strawberries, blackberries, using a jam made with the same fruit.

Makes 6–8 lollies, depending on the size of your mould

375g Greek yoghurt
180ml full-fat milk or single cream
4 tablespoons raspberry jam
350g fresh raspberries, washed
2 teaspoons vanilla extract
1 teaspoon fresh lavender flowers,
*   picked from their stalks and chopped*

Place all the ingredients (except for the lavender flowers) into a food processor and blend until silky smooth. Add the lavender flowers and stir in.

Pour into ice-lolly moulds and freeze overnight.

If necessary, run the moulds under warm water for a few seconds to release these deliciously grown-up lollies!

Lilac
Syringa vulgaris

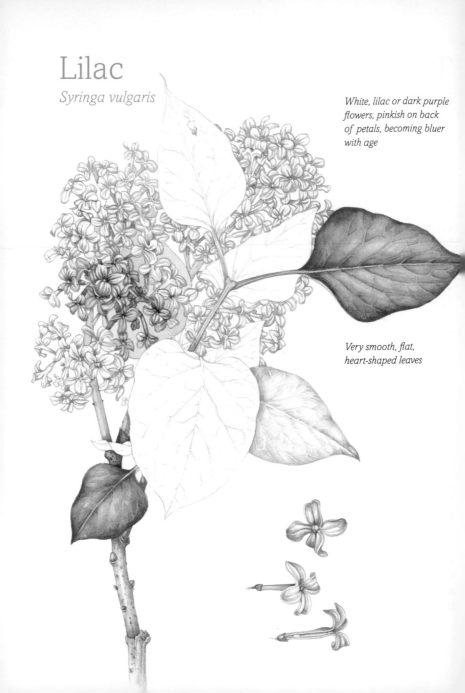

White, lilac or dark purple
flowers, pinkish on back
of petals, becoming bluer
with age

Very smooth, flat,
heart-shaped leaves

The lilac, like that other gorgeous edible garden plant, jasmine, and the olive, belongs to the *Oleaceae* family.

Lilacs are fully hardy and will withstand a good deal of frost and snow. They prefer to have their roots in deep, fertile soil that's well watered and well drained. They're deciduous, have heart-shaped leaves and, best of all, panicles of tiny, four-petalled, densely clustered flowers, ranging from a snowy white through to the deepest mauve and which smell absolutely glorious. Originating in the southern regions of Europe and in East Asia, the word lilac is derived from a Persian word meaning 'blue'; the genus name *Syringa* is from the Greek *syrinx*, referring to a hollow tube; the pith was at one time removed from the stem of the lilac to make a flute-like instrument.

In the Victorian era, a rumour sprang up that it was unlucky to bring lilac into the house. I picked this superstition up from my grandmother and was extremely disappointed when, as a child, I was told that I couldn't bring the lovely fragrant stems indoors. It's likely, however, that this superstition was seeded by housemaids who wouldn't want to add sweeping up dropped lilac flowers to the burden of dawn-to-dusk chores. The same superstition also applied to elderflower and maythorn blossoms, which, like lilac, are both small-flowered and heavily scented plants.

Medicinal Use

Lilac flowers, combined with the flowers of the linden tree, were used by the early European colonists of America to treat internal worms and parasites. A paste made of the flowers was reputed to soothe insect bites and stings. The plant was also used to prevent malaria; whether it worked or not has not yet been determined.

Culinary Use

Individual lilac flowers, removed from their stems, make a pretty, edible garnish, but to get the right flavour, you'd need to eat lots of them all together, which isn't particularly pleasant. The best way to use lilac is as an infusion or a subtle flavouring. For instance, you could add a handful of lilac flowers to double cream with a little white caster sugar and then refrigerate overnight for a lovely accompaniment to strawberries. If possible, it is best not to wash flowers too much, otherwise you can lose some of the pollen, which gives much of the flavour.

Jeff's Lilac Wine

Who hasn't heard the song 'Lilac Wine'? My favourite version is by Jeff Buckley and the recipe here is therefore named after him.

This wine needs to sit for a year to allow the dry, crisp flavours to develop before opening. Also it is quite fiddly – you need to pull each individual flower from the stalk, so engage willing friends around the kitchen table to help.

Makes 4 x 75cl bottles

*1 litre (in volume) individual lilac
    flowers*
*2 litres boiling water, plus extra for
    topping up the demijohn*
1kg white caster sugar
juice and zest of 2 unwaxed oranges
2 teaspoons dried yeast

Gather the flowers in the full heat of the sun for optimum flavour, rejecting any browning blossoms. Separate the individual blossoms and pack into a measuring jug to make 1 litre in volume. Put them into a food-grade bucket (preferably with a fitted lid). Pour the boiling water over them and add the sugar and the orange juice and zest. Leave to cool to blood temperature, then add the yeast, following the packet instructions. Cover and leave for 2 days. Strain the liquid into a demijohn, add an airlock and leave in a warm, dry, dark place at an even temperature for up to 16 weeks or until the bubbling of the fermentation stops.

Siphon the liquid into sterilised bottles, being careful to make sure that no sediment at the bottom of the demijohn goes into the bottle. Cork the bottles, and store in a dark place for 1 year, before opening and enjoying.

Lilac Meringue Pavlova

Makes 1 pavlova, serving 8

For the meringue
3 egg whites
60 individual lilac flowers, stems
  removed, plus extra for decoration
150g white granulated sugar

For the filling
150ml double cream
150ml Greek yoghurt
icing sugar, to taste (optional)
a handful of blueberries, or raspberries,
  or chopped strawberries (or a mixture
  of all three)
1 tablespoon lilac flowers, removed
  from their stems, plus extra for
  decoration

Preheat the oven to 140°C/gas 1 and line two 22 x 32cm baking trays with parchment paper.

To make the meringue, put the egg whites into a squeaky-clean bowl and whisk until stiff; if you're brave, try holding the bowl upside-down over your head to test if it's stiff enough.

Put the lilac flowers and sugar in a food processor and blitz for about 30 seconds just before using. Add the lilac sugar, a tablespoon at a time, to the egg whites, whisking again to stiff peaks. Then place a large oval-shaped dollop on to each of the prepared baking trays (you could of course make lots of smaller meringues if you prefer).

Bake for 1 hour, or a little longer if necessary, until the meringues are golden and lift easily from the parchment paper. Leave to cool completely.

To make the filling, whip the cream to just firm in a bowl. Add the yoghurt and sift in the icing sugar, if using. Add the fresh fruits and the lilac flowers and stir to combine. Place one of the meringues on a serving dish. Spread half the cream filling over the top and place the second meringue on top. Spread the rest of the topping over it and scatter with some lilac flowers.

Lilac Vodka

Makes 2 x 75cl bottles

9 fresh lilac heads
750ml vodka
500ml white caster sugar
250ml water

Note: *You will need a couple of 1-litre glass clip-top jars (e.g. Kilner jars) for this recipe.*

Wash the lilac heads and trim any stem and stalks. Put three of the lilac heads into a glass clip-top jar and pour in the vodka. Leave to soak for 6 hours, then strain the liquid from the flowers. Repeat twice more, using the strained vodka and three fresh flower heads each time.

While the last three flowers are soaking, put the sugar and water into a heavy-bottomed pan and heat until the sugar has dissolved.

Strain the vodka and return it to the jar along with the sugar syrup, and seal. Leave for a month before using.

Lindka's Lilac Cooler

For a cooling drink, put a couple of fresh lilac heads, removing as much of the stem as possible, into a 2-litre glass jug. Add some strongly scented red rose petals, honeysuckle flowers and sprigs of forget-me-not. Sprinkle a couple of tablespoons of white caster sugar over the flowers, then top with iced water. Leave to infuse for 15 minutes before drinking.

Candied Lilacs

This recipe may be time-consuming, but it's the sort of thing you can do while listening to a good radio play.

Makes 200g

100g white caster sugar
100g individual lilac flowers, stems
*   removed*
50ml water

In a mortar, grind 50g of the caster sugar to a very fine powder. (Do not use icing sugar as it contains a small volume of anti-caking agent which will interfere with the set of the sugar.) Wash the lilac flowers and leave to dry.

Line a baking tray with greaseproof paper and dust it with approximately a third of the ground caster sugar.

Put the 50g of unground caster sugar and the water in a pan and bring to the boil. Continue to cook, making sure the syrup doesn't burn, until a sugar thermometer reads 105°C, or use the cold saucer test (see page 13). Dip each flower into the syrup, one at a time, using tweezers, and place on the prepared baking tray. Repeat with the remaining flowers, then dust with another third of the ground sugar and leave in a cool place for 24 hours to dry completely.

Store in an airtight jar, layering the candied flowers with the remaining ground caster sugar.

Linden

Tilia

Heart-shaped leaves are highly shiny on top, matt and paler on underside

Small white flowers with open sepals, borne at an angle from papery base

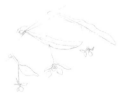

Tilia means 'broad-leafed' and the misleading 'lime' common name derives from the Middle-English word, *lind*, meaning 'flexible'. Found in all parts of the northern hemisphere including Asia, there are some 30 different species of linden tree.

Linden are deciduous and some species grow to a height of 40m. They like fertile, well-drained soils and will withstand cold temperatures but need plenty of rain. It's more likely that you'll see these beautiful trees in the grounds of stately homes or parks than in more humble domestic gardens; they were a favourite of the great Victorian landscape gardeners. Linden trees grow to a great age; specimens as old as 2,000 years and more have been recorded. In some towns lindens are also popular street trees, although if you were to park your car underneath one in the summer you might regret it, as the gloopy drops of sticky pollen that splash down from the blossoms are hard to remove from paintwork. Densely foliated, the canopy of this tree has abundant foliage in the summer, almost like a child's drawing of a tree. What makes the linden very special are its flowers; narrow bracts give forth a stem from which dangle the clusters of pretty small yellow blossoms with five petals that bloom in midsummer. Popular with both bees and their keepers, the honey made from linden flowers is said to be one of the best in the world. Butterflies and moths, too, love the linden, including the Lime Hawk-Moth, which is named after its favourite food. The tree's flowers have a delicate but distinctive floral scent which marries with their flavour; honey-like, slightly citrusy (more like oranges than lemons, though) and with a faint whiff of jasmine. It comes as no surprise that perfumiers use these blossoms in their scents; Jo Malone's 'French Lime Blossom' and Elizabeth Arden's '5th Avenue', for example.

In Germany it was once believed that the linden tree belonged to lovers. It was also a symbol of the truth and so any judicial meeting in which the truth of a matter needed to be determined was held beneath the tree.

Common Names

Basswood, lime tree, bee tree, whitewood, chocolate tree.

Medicinal Use

Linden has many and varied applications. During the First World War the flowers were used as a febrifuge – that is, to bring on a fever to help 'sweat out' infections. The flowers are used to cure ailments of the respiratory tract and in treating colds and flu. They are also used to treat high blood pressure and hypertension.

Culinary Use

Probably the simplest and best way to enjoy linden is to take a handful of the fresh new leaves (not the older ones) and make a sandwich of them with home-made bread, good-quality butter and a squeeze of fresh lemon juice.

The flowers make a wonderful tea, which the French call *tilleul*. Simply gather the flowers and infuse in boiling water for 5 minutes; drink with sugar or honey or without. It's lovely. I mean really, really delicious. You only need a cluster or two of the flowers per person and they can be used fresh or, better still, left to dry for 3 weeks. Drying the flowers increases the flavour and they can be stored in airtight containers. The leaves, too, can be cooked in the same way as any green vegetable, and their slight astringent taste rendered more palatable by steaming or by combining with other, milder-flavoured greens. The fruits of the tree – round, hard nut-like objects about 1cm in diameter – start to appear in late summer and early autumn. This fruit has a chocolate-like flavour, hence the common name 'chocolate tree'. If you want to try the recipes here, the fruits should be picked when they are young and still soft and green.

Linden Schnapps

This flavoured schnapps might be an acquired taste, so make a small amount to make sure you like the flavour – then make more if you do. Pick the flowers on a dry, sunny day when their flavour will be at its best. Do not wash or clean the flowers – you don't want to lose any of the pollen, which is what imparts the characteristic flavour of the plant.

Pick enough fresh linden flowers to fill a jar with a clip-top lid. Pour vodka over the blossoms, put on the lid and leave in a dark place at an even temperature for 3 days (no longer, otherwise you'll end up with a slightly musty taste). Strain the schnapps through a coffee filter paper to remove solids and fine debris, then decant into a sterilised bottle. Keep in the freezer and serve ice-cold, in shot glasses.

Linden Chocolate

Makes 500g

40g dried linden flowers
500g unripe green linden-tree fruits
a few drops of almond or grapeseed oil

Using a pestle and mortar, grind the dried flowers to as fine a powder as you can muster. Put the flower powder in a bowl and set aside.

Pound the fruits into a paste with a pestle and mortar or in a food processor. Mix this fruit paste with the powdered flowers and a drop or two of almond or grapeseed oil as necessary to make a thick but spreadable paste.

Serve spread on fresh bread or toast or use as a filling for a sponge cake. You could also make butterfly buns, using this unusual spread in place of cream.

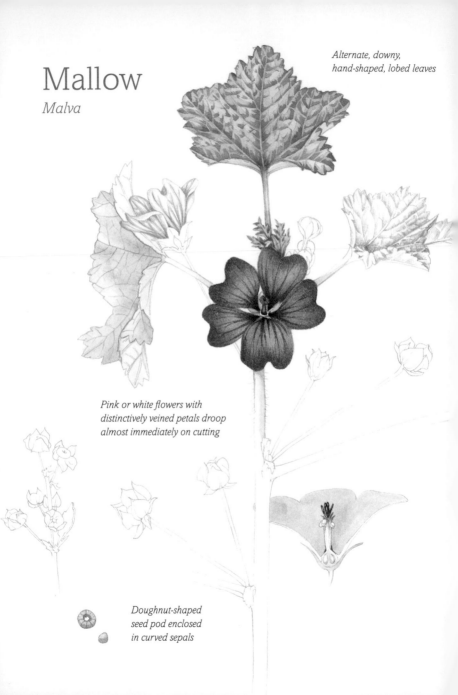

Mallow
Malva

Alternate, downy,
hand-shaped, lobed leaves

Pink or white flowers with
distinctively veined petals droop
almost immediately on cutting

Doughnut-shaped
seed pod enclosed
in curved sepals

There are some 25–30 different varieties of mallow, which you may occasionally find in the wild, although there are often garden escapes too (cultivated plants that have gone feral, as it were). You could plant your garden with a veritable rainbow of these fast-growing plants, which, in one season, given rich soil, full sun and plenty of water, will grow up to 3m high. They thrive in a range of conditions as well and although many gardening books advise that mallow won't survive a frost, from my experience if they are sheltered by a wall, they can survive temperatures of -10°C.

Native to Europe, Africa and Asia but naturalised in many other regions including the US, the name mallow comes from the Old English *malwe*, meaning 'soft'. The leaves, which are almost circular in shape with five lobes, do indeed have a fuzzy, downy feel to them. The flowers are approximately 5cm in diameter, with petals whose robustness belies their delicate appearance. Although in some parts of the world we've largely lost the habit of eating the mallow, the early Romans, Egyptians and Chinese included them in their diet on a regular basis and they are still used commonly in Greece, among other places. In fact, the mallow is one of the earliest recorded plants. Horace, the Roman poet (born 65 BC) wrote about it when describing his diet, saying (except in Latin, of course) something along the lines of, 'As for me, olives, endives and mallows provide sustenance enough.' The petals and seeds of the plant are also edible – the seeds are sometimes called cheeses. They taste sweet and nutty and make a nice nibble but are too fiddly for most of us to want to collect in any volume.

The *Malvaceae* family includes *Althaea officinalis*, whose mucilaginous roots were once used as the basis of a confection that you'll know better as the marshmallow, after the folk name of the plant. These days, you'd be hard-pressed to find marshmallow sweets that use the plant itself as an ingredient. Extracting the mucilage is time-consuming and difficult.

Common Names and Species

Cheese cake, pick cheese, billy buttons, bread and cheese, round dock, pancake plant (the last two, presumably, referring to the circular leaves), *M. sylvestris* (illustrated opposite).

Medicinal Use

The mucilaginous nature of the plant means that it has been used as a soothing throat tonic and there's an old Russian legend that underscores this use. A Tartar warlord, irritated by the persistent coughing of his son, swore that he would kill one child every day until the boy's cough was cured. The boy's sensible mother took some mallow roots, mashed them up and fed them to her son and, presto, the cough was cured.

Culinary Use

Mallow leaves can be eaten raw, but the slight furriness, which luckily disappears with cooking, might be off-putting. The leaves are mild-tasting and can be cooked in the same way as spinach. Pick young mallow leaves for cooking; the older ones get tough and stringy. To check that the leaves are good to use, pull the sides gently. If they stretch slightly before they tear, then they're fine.

Wilt them down and use in a pizza sauce to get some greens into your children. You can also use the larger of the young leaves to make *dolmades*.

Melokhia Soup

This recipe was given to me by Yolante Tsiabokalu, who was the first-ever female rapper in Greece and is a part of the Low Bap hip-hop collective. Mallows are a popular vegetable in Yolante's home country and she first cooked this using the abundance of mallow plants that had self-seeded in my garden.

Serves 6 as a starter, or 4 as a main course

6 garlic cloves, crushed
1 tablespoon olive oil
sea salt and freshly ground pepper,
   to taste
1 fresh red chilli, chopped
500g young mallow leaves
2 litres vegetable stock
1 tablespoon dried herbs of your
   choice, tied into a bouquet garni
juice of 1 lemon
250g Greek yoghurt (slightly watered
   down to make it thinner, if you wish),
   to serve

Fry the crushed garlic in the olive oil with a little salt. Add the chilli and mix into a paste.

Wash the mallow leaves and chop finely, using a mezzaluna if you have one, until you have a pulp.

In a large pan, bring the stock to a boil and add the mallow leaves. Boil for 10 minutes, then add the garlic and chilli paste, reduce the heat and cook for a further 10 minutes, stirring. Squeeze in the lemon juice just before serving. Because the mallow leaves are slightly mucilaginous, the soup will be thicker than you might expect and has a creamy texture.

Serve with a swirl of yoghurt and a sprinkle of salt and pepper.

Caramelised Onion, Feta and Mallow Pie

Serves 4–6

1 large potato, cut into chunks
a knob of butter, plus extra for greasing
1 tablespoon vegetable oil
3 medium red onions, thinly sliced
2 teaspoons granulated white sugar
½ tablespoon balsamic vinegar
a good handful of young mallow
    leaves, blanched for a few seconds
    and chopped
1 tablespoon cream
salt and pepper, to taste
200g feta cheese, crumbled
a sprig of thyme leaves, chopped
500g ready-made puff pastry
1 egg, beaten, for the egg wash

Preheat the oven to 180°C/gas 4. Grease a 25cm pie dish.

Cook the potato in boiling salted water until tender enough to be mashed. Leave to cool.

Heat the butter and vegetable oil in a heavy-bottomed pan. Add the onions and cook, stirring, until golden, then add the sugar and balsamic vinegar. Keep stirring until the onions start to caramelise, then add the blanched and chopped mallow leaves. Remove from the heat and cover.

Mash the potato with the cream, season well and stir in the feta, mallow mixture and thyme leaves.

Cut the pastry in half and, on a lightly floured surface, roll each half to a circle about 3mm thick. Line the pie dish with one circle of pastry – don't worry if the pastry overhangs the dish.

Spoon all the ingredients into the pie dish and cover the pie with the remaining pastry. Seal the edges with water and trim off any excess pastry.

Brush the top of the pie with the beaten egg and cut three small holes in the pastry lid with a sharp knife, to allow the steam to escape.

Cook for 35 minutes or until golden – turn halfway through to ensure an even finish.

Leave to cool for 5 minutes before serving with a crisp salad.

Mulberry

Morus

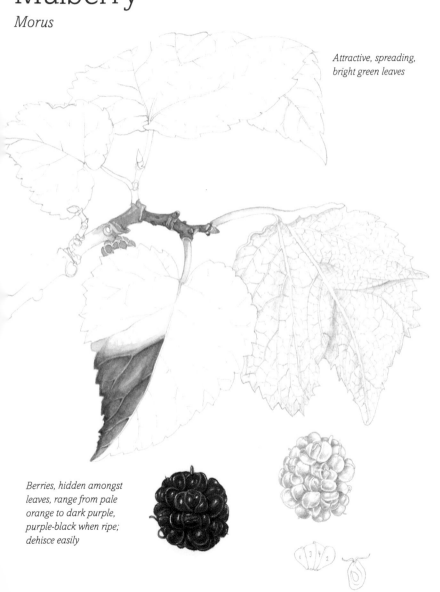

Attractive, spreading,
bright green leaves

Berries, hidden amongst
leaves, range from pale
orange to dark purple,
purple-black when ripe;
dehisce easily

The best-known fact about mulberries is probably that the leaves are the only thing that silkworms will eat and so the plant is essential to the production of the fabric. In fact, in the early 17th century, King James 1 was so keen to establish a silk trade in England that he issued an edict encouraging the trees to be cultivated; however, he mistakenly handed out seeds of the black mulberry rather than the white, which is indigenous to Asia, so sadly the production of silk in the UK was hampered at that time.

There are 16 or so species of mulberry growing all over the northern hemisphere from the Himalayas to the Americas. The mulberry is a hardy tree, preferring a nutritious soil that's slightly on the damp side, but not minding whether it is in sun or shade. Remarkably easy to propagate by cuttings, the young mulberry tree grows so fast in its early years that you can practically see it shooting up, although it slows down after five years or so. It will reach a maximum height of 15m. In some places, the lovely mulberry is seen as a pest because it sends out suckers and is virtually indestructible, so if you decide to get one for your garden, beware. The leaves are a little like beech leaves, pale green and with serrated edges; the fruits vary in colour according to the variety, but the berries of the black mulberry (*M. nigra*), illustrated here, are said to be the tastiest of all. The berries look like fatter, elongated versions of blackberries and the juice will stain your lips and fingers and everything else a luscious purple colour that is difficult to remove from fabric.

The species name for the plant is *Morus*, after the Greek god Moros, whose role it was to drive human mortals towards their destiny; the equivalent Roman god was Fatus, meaning 'fate'. *Moros* means 'doom' and is the root of the word 'morose'. In the Greek legend of the doomed lovers Pyramus and Thisbe, the couple arrange to meet underneath a white mulberry tree and, in a plot which Shakespeare must surely have appropriated for Romeo and Juliet, Pyramus mistakenly believes that his love, Thisbe, has been killed by a lion and so ends his own life by falling on his sword; the fruits of the tree, originally white, turn red with spattered blood. Thisbe discovers the body and she, too, kills herself by the same means. The gods turned the fruit of the tree red in their honour.

Common Species
M. nigra, M. alba, M. rubra.

Medicinal Use
As a medicine, the mulberry is a useful plant. Traditionally, the berries

were made into a syrup which has both laxative and expectorant qualities. The bark of the black mulberry was used to treat tapeworm in both animals and humans. Latterly, the American Diabetes Association discovered that the leaves can help regulate blood sugar levels and use of the plant in type 2 diabetes is being investigated.

Culinary Use

All mulberries are edible. The young, unopened leaves, too, can be eaten in the same way as any green vegetable. For a substantial side dish, boil the leaves for 20 minutes, add fried onions and garlic, top with cheese and brown under the grill. It's the berries though, generally abundant, which are the stars of the show.

Mulberry White Rum

Makes 750ml

450g ripe mulberries
700ml white rum
150g white caster sugar
100g roasted hazelnuts

Pick over and wash the mulberries. Then simply put all the ingredients into a large glass jar (or jars) with a clip-top lid and leave in a cool, dark place for 2–3 months, shaking it occasionally during the first week so that the sugar dissolves completely.

Strain the rum through a sieve to remove the berries and the nuts (the soaked mulberries can be used in a fruit crumble and the nuts added to the crumble topping). Then strain the rum again, if necessary, through muslin to remove any further debris. Decant into a sterilised 750ml bottle.

Mulberry and Lavender Cheesecake

Serves 6–8

250g digestive biscuits, crushed
100g unsalted butter, melted, plus extra
for greasing
600g cream cheese
100g icing sugar, sifted, plus 25g for the
cheesecake topping
5 drops of lavender essence
200ml double cream
400g ripe mulberries
fresh lavender flowers, for decoration

Grease a 23cm loose-bottomed cake tin and line it with parchment paper.

Put the crushed biscuits in a bowl and pour in the melted butter. Stir until all the biscuits are well coated, then spoon the mixture into the prepared cake tin. Spread the mixture evenly over the bottom of the tin and press it down well. Refrigerate for 1 hour to set the base.

Put the cream cheese, the 100g of icing sugar and the lavender essence into a bowl and beat with a wooden spoon (or use an electric mixer) until smooth. Add the double cream and beat well. Spoon the mixture on to the cheesecake base and chill overnight.

Remove the cheesecake carefully from the tin and on to a serving dish.

Put half the mulberries into a food processor, add the 25g of icing sugar and a little water. Blend for 1 minute, then pass the fruit purée through a fine-meshed sieve to remove as many of the seeds as possible. Arrange the remaining mulberries on top of the cake and pour the purée over the top. Decorate with fresh lavender flowers.

Mulberry Floc

Based on a recipe from Gascony which traditionally uses raspberries, this is a delicious cross between a dessert and a liqueur, served after coffee.

Serves 6–8

500g mulberries
200g white caster sugar
½ bottle (375ml) of good red wine
2 tablespoons Armagnac

Pick over and wash the mulberries, then put them into a bowl and sprinkle the sugar over the top. Cover and leave overnight at room temperature to let the sugar draw the juices out of the berries.

Stir in the wine and the Armagnac, cover and leave overnight at room temperature once again to allow the flavours to blend together beautifully. Chill for a couple of hours before serving in wine goblets.

Nasturtium

Tropaeolum

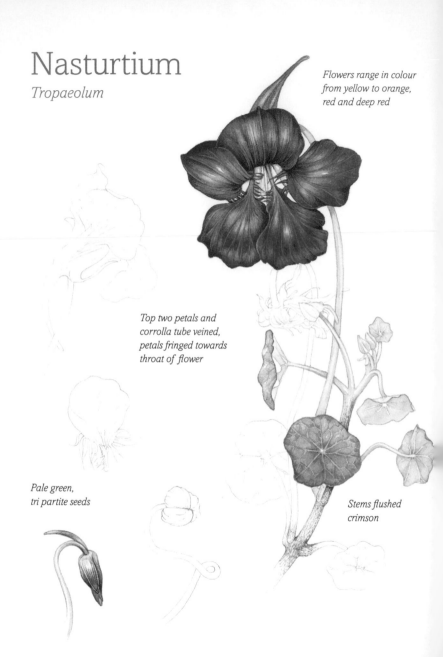

Flowers range in colour from yellow to orange, red and deep red

Top two petals and corolla tube veined, petals fringed towards throat of flower

Pale green, tri partite seeds

Stems flushed crimson

Strictly speaking, a nasturtium actually refers to a genus of watercress. For many of us, nasturtiums are probably the first plant that comes to mind when thinking of edible garden plants. And although the tropaeolum is not related to the watercress, nasturtiums, with their bright orange or yellow flowers, do contain an oil that is very similar to that found in the watercress, hence perhaps the confusion with the names. If you're ever nibbled on its leaves, flowers, seed heads or buds, you'll know the spicy, peppery taste very well; it's this flavour that gives the name nasturtium, from the Latin, *nasus tortus*, meaning 'nose twister', which is a pretty accurate description of the pungency of the flavour.

Although the bright fiery orange flowers are probably the ones we see most often, nasturtium blooms come in a wide range of colours including creamy whites, yellows, reds and a lovely purple-black. They have five petals and a distinctive little spur at the back of the flower in which pollen collects. The blossoms are borne singly on short stalks and are prolific. The leaves are very distinctive, too, looking rather like flowers themselves, being a circular shape with a ray of veins radiating out from the centre.

Nasturtiums were introduced into Europe in the 18th century by the great Swedish botanist, Linnaeus. He named them tropaeolum after the rather grizzly Roman custom of erecting a pole topped by a trophy (*tropaeum* in Latin) in the form of the armour and other effects of the slain enemy. Linnaeus said that the flowers reminded him of bloodstained helmets, and the leaves, the shields of the dead soldiers. The French, German, Italian and Spanish names for the plant all derive from the Italian word *cappuccio*, meaning 'hood', which refers to the shape of the flower itself.

Native to South America and Chile where the flowers enjoy hot, dry conditions, nasturtiums will grow happily in poor soil with little moisture; in fact, give them too rich a soil and too moist an environment and your nasturtiums will tend to produce fewer flowers in favour of leaves. They're not happy sitting in puddles of water for any length of time. Some nasturtiums tend to trail and some have a climbing or tumbling habit and there are also varieties that look more like little shrubs. They're great plants for children to begin gardening with since the seeds are large and satisfying for small hands and they very rarely fail to produce an impressive crop so long as the seeds are planted once the danger of frost has passed.

Medicinal Use

Nasturtium is rich in vitamin C, which explains why it was once used to prevent scurvy. More curiously, as a folk remedy, the plant was used to prevent baldness; the hot mustardy juice, which can be extracted from the plant, was believed to stimulate the hair follicles. Even today, some practitioners will treat balding heads with a mashed-up poultice of nasturtium leaves and flowers, although there is no conclusive evidence that this will have the desired effect.

Culinary Use

The leaves, flowers buds and young seeds of nasturtium are all piquantly peppery. The leaves, buds and stems are crisp and chewy in texture while the flowers are soft. All parts of the nasturtium can be eaten raw and they make a colourful addition to salad, although a little of that peppery taste does go a long way. An unusual way to present the flowers is to stuff them with a mixture of cream cheese, chives or mint; the cool flavour of the soft cheese offsets the mustardy tang of the petals very nicely. This makes a good starter for a summer supper party, even if it's something of a 70s throwback. Nasturtium flowers stuffed with vanilla ice-cream works well, too.

Nasturtium-Leaf Soup

This recipe is in honour of Dwight Eisenhower, the 34th President of the US. He loved his nasturtiums and devised a soup made from them.

Serves 4–6

a knob of butter
1 tablespoon vegetable oil
2 medium red onions, finely chopped
3 medium potatoes, chopped
25–30 nasturtium leaves, washed
1 litre stock
300ml single cream, plus extra to serve
sea salt and freshly ground pepper, to taste
celery salt, to taste, to serve
nasturtium leaves and flowers, for decoration

Melt the butter and oil in a heavy-bottomed pan, then add the onions and cook, stirring, until golden. Add the potatoes and the nasturtium leaves and stir until the leaves are wilted and the potatoes are beginning to brown.

Add the stock and stir in the cream, then season well with sea salt and pepper and simmer for 20 minutes. Blend the soup with a stick blender or in a food processor. Serve with a swirl of cream and a pinch of celery salt and decorate each bowl with a nasturtium leaf and flower.

Pickled Nasturtium Seed Pods

Often described as a substitute for capers, these pickled seed pods don't really taste like capers, to me, but they do add exactly the same sort of 'kick' where it's needed, in pasta or pizza sauces, in salads, or added to bread dough. If you have an abundance of nasturtiums, then picking the seed pods seems to make more seeds form even faster! However, don't bother using anything but the young, tender seed pods for this recipe and remove any that are showing signs of mould and insect activity, etc.

Makes enough to fill 1 x 230g jar

15g salt
300ml boiling water
100g fresh nasturtium seed pods, stems
    removed
fresh herbs of your choice
5 black peppercorns
1–2 small fresh red chillies (optional)
200ml white wine vinegar

Put the salt into a bowl, add the boiling water and stir to dissolve the salt. Leave to cool and then add the nasturtium pods and leave for 24 hours. Drain and dry the pods thoroughly.

Put the herbs, peppercorns and chillies, if using, into a sterilised jar and add the nasturtium pods, filling the jar to 1cm from the top. Pour the vinegar into the jar. Make sure the seeds are completely covered with vinegar. Seal the jar and leave for 3 weeks before opening. Refrigerate after opening and keep the seeds immersed in the vinegar, and the pickle will keep for one year.

Nasturtium Pesto

Some recipes for nasturtium pesto recommend that you cook the nasturtium first, but I find that this isn't necessary. You can use just nasturtium leaves if you want, but I would advise combining them with a milder leaf – if you happen to have any sedum (see page 184), its cool juiciness works a treat with the hot pepperiness of the nasturtiums. You could also use ground elder, mint and hosta leaves in this recipe.

Serves 6–8 as a side dish

1 packed mugful nasturtium leaves
¼ mugful roughly chopped nuts
  (pine nuts, blanched almonds,
  walnuts, even peanuts)
¼ mugful roughly grated mature
  hard cheese
2 tablespoons good-quality olive oil
fresh lemon juice, to taste
sea salt, to taste

Wash and dry the nasturtium leaves and chop them roughly. Put the leaves, nuts and cheese into a food processor or blender, add 1 tablespoon of the olive oil and blend until just combined. (If you don't have a food processor or blender, chop the leaves finely with a knife or mezzaluna – a curved, two-handled knife – and add to the chopped nuts and grated cheese.)

Add more oil to loosen the pesto as necessary. Transfer to a bowl, stir in the lemon juice and add sea salt to taste. Stir again, then add a little more olive oil to cover the ingredients. Store in a clean, lidded jar or a bowl in the fridge. Bring to room temperature before using.

Oregon Grape

Mahonia aquifolium

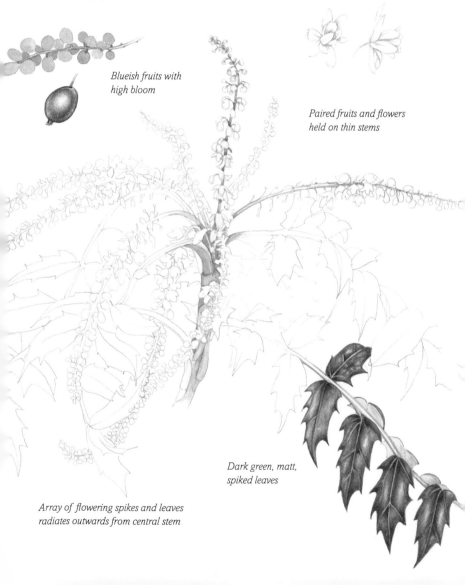

Blueish fruits with
high bloom

Paired fruits and flowers
held on thin stems

Dark green, matt,
spiked leaves

Array of flowering spikes and leaves
radiates outwards from central stem

If you're American, you will know this plant by its common name. In the UK, however, the plant is called *Mahonia aquifolium*, named after the horticulturalist Bernard McMahon, who found it in North America when he was a part of the Lewis and Clark expedition of 1804. Indeed, the Oregon grape is the symbolic flower of the US state of Oregon. *Aquifolium* means 'holly-leaved'. The Oregon grape is native to Asia and the Himalayas as well as the Americas and there are some 70 species of the plant, which belongs to the same family as the berberis (see page 41).

The beauty of the Oregon grape often goes unnoticed since, as a spiky evergreen, it is a popular plant for rather dull municipal planting schemes. Left unpruned, it will grow to a height of 2m and a width of about 1.5m. It doesn't seem to mind what kind of soil it grows in, or whether it is in sun or shade. But the yellow racemes of flowers smell sensational; what's even better is that the scent is at its best during the drab months of late winter, before spring. If you're parking somewhere in a city in early spring and you notice a beautiful honey-like perfume, there's a good chance that the scent is coming from the humble, spiky plants that surround the concrete lots. What's more, the berries that follow the blossoms are not only edible, but rich in vitamin C, too. Their natural sharpness needs to be tempered with some sweetness and you do need quite a few berries to make anything worthwhile. But the fact that local councils buy them in their thousands for urban landscaping means the berries are perfect for foraging.

Common Names
Mahonia, mountain grape, holly-leaved barberry.

Medicinal Use
Some Native American tribes used the berries to treat indigestion and loss of appetite, and today the mahonia is used by herbalists to treat digestive ailments, including gastritis. An active ingredient in the berry, called berberine, stimulates bile secretions. Extracts of mahonia can also help the absorption of vitamins and minerals in foods. It is also used against eye infections.

Culinary Use
The early colonists in Amercia made much use of the ripe and plump berries, which have a sharply acidic flavour, and discovered that the dark blue ones tasted the best. Wear protective clothing and gloves when harvesting the berries, to guard against those prickles. The juice of the ripe berries will also stain clothes and utensils. They are high in pectin,

so lend themselves well to jams and preserves. The berry contains a small seed, which can be removed by passing the fruit through a sieve. Mahonia flowers can be eaten raw or made into a lemonade-like drink.

Oregon-Grape Flower Lemonade

Makes 2 litres

2 handfuls of Oregon-grape flowers
500g white caster sugar
2 litres boiling water
zest and juice of 4 unwaxed lemons

Pick over the mahonia flowers, removing the stems, and wash them.

Put the sugar in a heatproof jug and pour the boiling water over it. Stir until the sugar has dissolved. Leave to cool for 30 minutes, then add the lemon zest and juice and the flowers. Stir, then cover and leave overnight. Serve over ice.

Oregon-Grape Preserve

This works well with cheeses and meats, wherever a sweetly sour taste is called for. Try adding a few chillies if you like.

Makes 1 x 450g jar

500g (or more) Oregon grape berries
golden caster sugar (see method for
*   amount)*
fresh chillies, chopped, to taste
*   (optional)*
lemon juice (see method for amount)

Pick as many berries as you can harvest – 500g or more makes the effort worthwhile.

Wash them, pick over and remove any debris. Put the berries in a large pan and just cover with water. Boil for about 15 minutes, then press the mixture through a large sieve, in batches, to remove the seeds. Retain as much pulp as you can.

Weigh the resulting fruit pulp, then weigh out the same amount of caster sugar. Return the fruit pulp to the pan and bring to the boil, then add the sugar a little at a time, tasting as you go. Add the chillies, if using, to taste. Boil for a further 5 minutes, then remove from the heat. Leave to cool and add the fresh juice of 1 whole lemon for every 500g/2½ cups of berries.

Ladle the preserve into warm, sterilised jars and leave to cool before sealing with waxed discs and lids.

Oregon-Grape Jelly

This sweet jelly, with a hint of tartness, delivers the same sort of kick as marmalade. It's delicious spread on toast or served with a strong cheese.

Makes enough to fill 3 x 250ml jars

For the grape juice
500g Oregon-grape berries

For the jelly
*500ml Oregon-grape juice, made from
    above berries*
400ml golden caster sugar

Pick over the berries and rinse them. Put the berries in a pan and add half their volume of water. Cover and simmer for about 10 minutes or until the berries are soft. Mash the berries in the pan, using a potato masher, to release as much of their juice as possible. Put the fruit pulp in a jelly bag set over a bowl and leave to drip, preferably overnight.

The next day, pour the resulting juice into a large, non-reactive pan and cook to reduce by about a fifth. Add the sugar and cook over a medium heat, stirring to dissolve the sugar. Turn up the heat and bring to the boil, skimming away any scum which might form on the surface. If you have a sugar thermometer, heat the mixture to 105°C, or use the cold saucer test (see page 13) to check if it has reached setting point.

Pour into warm, sterilised jars. Once the jelly is cold, seal with waxed discs and put on the lids.

Passion Flower

Passiflora

Bright green, hand-shaped,
five-lobed, glabrous leaves

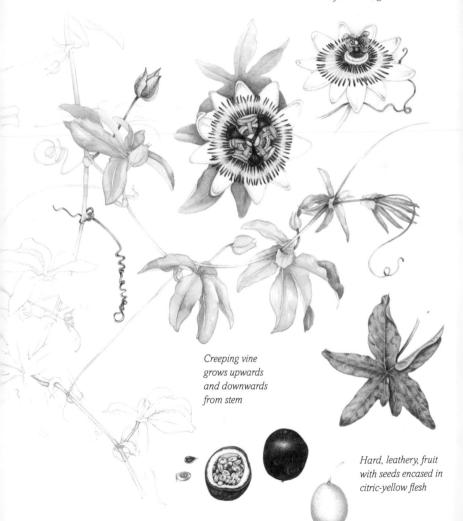

Creeping vine
grows upwards
and downwards
from stem

Hard, leathery, fruit
with seeds encased in
citric-yellow flesh

The fruit of this plant goes by too many different names to list them all here. For example, in Indonesia it's *markisa*, in Hawai *lilkoi* and in the UK and most English-speaking countries it's simply called passionfruit. It is also called maypop, granadilla and wild apricot.

The passion flower is a climbing plant which will reach a sprawl of up to 9m. They also grow fast and in the right circumstances can reach this sort of size in a single season. Native to the jungles of South America, the passion flower likes pretty much any kind of soil so long as it's well drained. Sunshine and heat are essential for this plant to thrive − a south-facing wall is a good spot or, in colder climates, a conservatory or greenhouse would be the best bet. However, if you cut the plant down to the base in the autumn and cover it with hessian and soil so it doesn't freeze, it will come back the following year. The plants are widely available; even supermarkets sell passion-flower plants for very little money. In fact, just three or four of the fruits, bought in the same supermarket, will generally cost more than the plant itself!

Those flowers are incredibly exotic-looking; there's something of a space-age insect about their design, or perhaps something from the imagination of Salvador Dali. The name comes from the Spanish missionary explorers who discovered the plant in the early 16th century; they believed that its features were symbolic of the Passion of Christ, its presence indicating God's seal of approval of their quest to tame the heathen jungle savages by introducing them to Christianity.

It's likely that they used the flower to tell the story of Christ, too. The sharp, pointed tips of the leaves, said the Spanish missionaries, represented the lance that was used to pierce Christ's side and the long, curling tendrils were the whips that lashed him. The ten petals represented the ten disciples who were loyal − missing out Judas Iscariot, the betrayer, and Peter, who denied Christ. The distinctive rays of tiny filaments represented the crown of thorns. The central ovary, with its indentation, represents the chalice and the three stigmata, the three nails in Christ's hands and feet; the five anthers are the number of wounds sustained. Hence, passion flower.

The flowers come in many different colours, but they are most commonly blue and white. And there's even more symbolic meaning here; those colours represent purity and heaven. The *P. edulis* variety sometimes goes by the name of granadilla, but this is nothing to do with the liqueur grenadine, which is actually made from pomegranates.

It's the passion-flower fruit which is edible – indeed delicious. Restricting root growth will help encourage a good yield of the fruits. In warmer climes, it is possible to get the plants to fruit infinitely, even in the UK, without the need for glass protection.

As well as the species mentioned here, there are several other edible types of passion fruit, so if you have one, check to see what it is.

Common Names and Species
Maypop, granadilla, wild apricot, and many more, *P. caerulea* (see illustration on page 172), *P. incarnata*.

Medicinal Use
Medicinally, passiflora is used to help people sleep and to allay nervous anxiety. It has a calming effect, and the extract is being studied for possible use in cases of ADHD.

Culinary Use
Passion fruits are at their sweetest and best when the skin has wrinkled a bit. To harvest the delicious sweet orangey flavour of the passion fruit, cut the fruit in half and scoop out the flesh. The distinctive black seeds are edible but if you prefer not to eat them, simply press the flesh through a fine-meshed sieve.

Use to top meringues, pour over ice-cream, or mix into a glass of prosecco.

Old Barn Tea Room Passion Cake

This recipe came to me via the Old Barn Tea Room in Torpantau, in the Brecon Beacons. The portions at the tea room are so generous that one cake would probably serve only 4; at home, though, the cake will serve about 10.

Serves 10

For the sponge
300g self-raising flour
1 teaspoon baking powder
50g desiccated coconut
1 teaspoon cinnamon
300g golden caster sugar
2 eggs, beaten, plus 2 egg whites
2 small ripe bananas, mashed
140g carrots, grated
432g tin lychees in their juice, fruit crushed and juice retained
150ml vegetable oil, plus extra for greasing

For the syrup
4 ripe passion fruit
lychee juice (from above tin)
25g golden caster sugar

For the filling
200g tub marscapone
100g butter, at room temperature
85g icing sugar, sifted
1 teaspoon rose extract

Preheat the oven to 180°C/gas 4. Grease three 20cm sandwich tins and line with parchment paper.

To make the sponge, sift the flour, baking powder, coconut, cinnamon and half the sugar into a large bowl and mix to combine.

In a separate bowl, mix together the 2 whole eggs, the banana, the grated carrot, the drained, crushed lychees and the oil.

In a clean bowl, beat the egg whites until stiff, then add the rest of the sugar and beat until stiff and glossy.

Add the fruit mixture to the flour mixture and stir until smooth, then fold in the egg whites. Divide the mixture between the prepared sandwich tins, smoothing with a palette knife, and bake for 25 minutes or until an inserted skewer comes out clean. Halfway through the baking time, swap the position of the tins in the oven to ensure that the cakes are all baked evenly. Leave the cakes to cool in their tins for 10 minutes, then transfer to a wire tray to cool completely.

To make the syrup, cut the passion fruit in half and scoop out the flesh and pips into a small pan. Add the lychee juice and the sugar and heat, bubbling, for about 10 minutes or until you have a thick, syrupy consistency.

To make the filling, mix together the marscapone and the butter until smooth, then beat in the sifted icing sugar and the rose extract. Cover and refrigerate.

Prick two of the cakes evenly with a skewer and drizzle the syrup equally over them, reserving some for the top of the cake. Spread the two cakes with the icing and stack all three together. Drizzle the remaining syrup over the top of the cake.

Rose

Rosa

Bushy foliage, with glossy, bright green, opposite leaves

Hips start flushed like apples, becoming scarlet when ripe

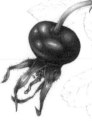

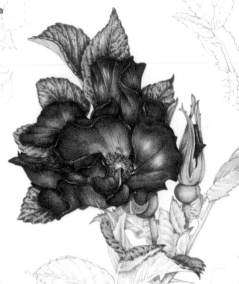

Moss-rose, cherry-red and rich purple flowers; ochre anthers producing cream pollen

Long, green thorns, absent on stipules

Does this plant need any further introduction? The rose is a favourite flower of many and there are over 100 species to choose from; different species hybridise with one another very readily, hence the astonishing variety. Roses come in just about all colours, from snowy white to a dark purple-black. They grow as bushes, or they can trail, or climb, or can be pruned into standard shapes. Miniature roses in pots are small enough to grace a dinner table. The wild rose has pale pink flowers tumbling through hedgerows; cultivated, long-stemmed red roses are the ultimate expression of love and come with a high price attached. And our love of roses is nothing new. We know that they were prized in Persia at least as far back as 500 BC, and fossilised roses tell us that they were on this planet some 35 million years ago.

If you want roses to grow in your garden, you can plant them in any kind of soil so long as you dig in plenty of nutrients and supply a regular plant feed. For the most part they prefer an open, sunny aspect, although the climbing varieties will happily scramble up trees. If you have a dead tree in your garden, rather than cutting it down, as rotting wood is a godsend for insects, why not plant a vigorous rambling rose at its base instead. The tree will look lovely covered in the blossoms.

Rosa canina, by the way, the common wild rose, which also goes under the name of dog rose, is so called because it was once believed to cure a person who'd had the misfortune to be bitten by a rabid dog.

Medicinal Use

Sometimes, old wives' tales about plants are proven to be true. Rosehip syrup has been used against colds and flu for generations and, indeed, it's been proven that the fruits contain a healthy dose of vitamin C, a discovery made as recently as the 1930s. Otherwise, Native Americans used every bit of the rose as a cure for a range of illnesses, including influenza, stomach upsets and fevers. The beautifully scented oil of roses, too, is used in aromatherapy to lift the spirits and to heal the grief of separation.

Culinary Use

Roses are not just beautiful, they are edible, too. The petals, leaves and hips of all roses can be used. To be fair, the only use I have found for the leaves is as a tea; simply infuse the fresh or dried leaves in water. Roseleaf tea is rich in tannin and while it does have a flavour of black tea, to be honest it's nothing to write home about. Rose petals and rosehips, however, are a different matter.

The rose illustrated here is the Chinese rose, *Rosa rugosa*, often used in municipal planting schemes in towns and cities, where the rich red bounty of the hips tends to be overlooked by busy shoppers.

Those large hips, the size of cherry tomatoes or sometimes even bigger, are so much easier to deseed than the smaller ones. Slice from top to bottom along one side with a scalpel, and put the hips into the freezer overnight. The next day, slice the fruit in half and the fuzzy seeds will pop out easily with the help of the pointed end of a knife. The seeds of all rosehips will irritate your throat and so need to be removed (school children also used them as an itching powder). As a perfume, the exotic, heady scented oil of roses, undiluted, is worth, in weight, more than gold.

With the first two basic syrup recipes below, one for rosehips, the other for rose petals, you can make a range of different dishes.

Rosehip Syrup

Makes 1.5 litres

1kg rosehips, seeds removed
3 litres boiling water
450g golden caster sugar

Pick over the hips and discard any less than perfect ones. Wash the hips thoroughly (rosehips tend to hold dust). Top and tail the rosehips – snip off the stalks and any fuzz at the top.

Put the hips into a heavy-bottomed pan and pour in the boiling water. Break up the hips by mashing with a potato masher, then bring back to the boil and simmer for 20 minutes. Remove from the heat, leave to cool, then pour the pulp into a jelly bag placed over a bowl. Leave to drip, preferably overnight.

The next day, put the resulting rosehip juice in the fridge. Add the pulp to a heavy-bottomed pan, and repeat the above step to make a second batch of juice.

When the juice is ready, measure 1.5 litres of water into the pan and make a note of where this comes up to. Pour all the rosehip juice into the pan, add the sugar and bring to the boil, cooking until the liquid has reduced down to the 1.5 litres mark. Leave to cool completely, then pour into sterilised bottles.

Rose-Petal Syrup

Makes about 350ml

250g fresh rose petals, washed if
necessary (the deeper the colour
of the petal, the deeper the
colour of the syrup)
200g golden granulated sugar
750ml boiling water
juice of 1 large unwaxed orange.

Place the rose petals in a non-reactive bowl. Add 50g of the sugar and rub the petals gently into the sugar, breaking them a little to release the oils (your fingers will smell gorgeous after this!). Cover with cling film and leave overnight.

The next day, put the rest of the sugar and the boiling water into a pan and heat gently to dissolve the sugar. Add the rose-petal and sugar mixture, then bring slowly to a gentle simmer and cook for about 30 minutes, or until a sugar thermometer reads 105°C. The liquid will have reduced by approximately a half. Remove from the heat and allow to cool. When it has cooled, strain the syrup into a bowl and add the orange juice. Pour into a clean, sterilised bottle or other container and freeze, if you wish.

Rose-Petal and Orange Kulfi

Serves 4–6

600ml full-fat milk
300ml condensed milk
100ml rose syrup (see recipe opposite)
2 handfuls of strongly scented rose
petals, washed if necessary, torn into
small pieces
½ teaspoon cinnamon powder
(optional)
2 tablespoons chopped pistachios or
macadamia nuts

Pour the full-fat and condensed milks into a heavy-bottomed pan and bring to the boil. Cook to reduce it to just over a third of its original volume, then remove from the heat and leave to cool, uncovered. Once cooled, add the rose syrup, the petals and the cinnamon, if using, stirring well. Then either churn in an ice-cream maker, according to the manufacturer's instructions, or pour into a freezer container and freeze for a couple of hours, then break up the surface with a fork and apply a stick blender, for a lovely smooth consistency. Return to the freezer for another couple of hours. Take the kulfi out of the freezer about 15 minutes before serving with a sprinkling of chopped nuts.

Rosehip Sweets

This recipe shows just how brilliant *Rosa rugosa* hips are for using in a variety of dishes.

Serves 6–8

150g granulated white sugar
200g Rosa rugosa *rosehips*
1 tablespoon water
2 tablespoons lemon juice

Line a baking tray with parchment paper and cover it with 75g granulated sugar.

Prepare the rosehips, as described on page 178, to remove all traces of seeds.

In a non-reactive pan, dissolve the remaining sugar in the water and lemon juice, add the rosehips and turn them gently until they're coated in the syrup; tilt the pan from side to side, shaking it occasionally to ensure good coverage and to prevent burning.

Remove the hips to the prepared baking tray. Roll the hips in the sugar to coat them; at this point you will have a gooey mess! Leave to dry in a cool place or eat immediately, with ice-cream.

You can also stir these sugar-coated hips into a muffin mix to make rosehip muffins, or, similarly, add to sponge cake, stirring the hips through the batter at the end of the mixing.

Rose-Petal Gin

Makes 75cl

1 x 75cl bottle of gin
3 tablespoons sugar
a large handful of strongly scented rose petals, washed if necessary

Pour the gin into a clean, wide-necked bottle or other container. Add the sugar and enough rose petals to fill up the bottle or container, leaving a gap of 2cm at the top to allow you to shake the bottle. Leave for about 6 hours, shaking and tasting occasionally to check the flavour as it develops, then strain the gin to remove the petals, and decant into a sterilised bottle.

Sea Holly

Eryngium

Powdery-blue thistle-like
flower head

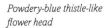

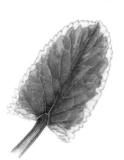

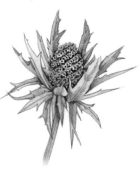

Spiny, glabrous,
silvery-grey, sometimes
variegated leaves

Tall, fleshy plant

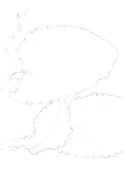

As the name suggests, sea holly is a plant with very spiny leaves, a bit like holly leaves, with silvery-grey foliage and stems and a divinely coloured powdery-blue thistle-like flower head. The one illustrated here is a particularly pretty variegated type.

Although sea holly started out life as a maritime plant, growing wild in coastal regions around the UK, the plant has gained status in more recent years as a sculptural addition to ornamental gardens and the thought of actually eating the thing, I would guess, is a long way off anyone's agenda, especially given all those spikes.

Sea holly grows to approximately 50cm tall, preferring dry soil, and is happy, as you'd imagine, growing in salty areas. The name has Greek origins and means 'to stop belching' and was once used as a cure for gassiness. The lovely blue flowers appear in mid-summer and the plant prefers full sun.

Medicinal Use

As a medicine, sea holly has many uses beyond the instruction given by Culpeper, who advised, 'The distilled water of the whole herb, when the leaves and stalks are young, is profitably drank for all the purposes aforesaid, and helps the melancholy of the heart, and is available in quartin and quotidian agues; as also for

them that have their necks drawn awry, and cannot turn them without turning their whole body.'

Latterly, it is used in treatments of the liver and kidneys, to treat enlargement of the prostate gland, as well as to relieve persistent and painful coughing. Colchester, in Essex, was at one time renowned for its candied eryngo roots, which were not just a confection but, reputedly, a remedy for coughs and colds as well as being an aphrodisiac.

Culinary Use

I kept coming across 'eryngoes', using the roots of the plant, in old cookery books; in days gone by it seems they were a popular edible plant, and since I have a fairly decent stand of them in my garden, seemingly growing out of rubble substrate but originally bought about 15 years ago from a garden centre, I thought I'd give them a go. You can tell just how much sea holly must have grown in coastal areas at one time by looking at the volumes of roots that are stated in old recipes – for example, eyringo conserve, which requires 1lb (almost 500g) of roots, but then the root system of the plant does extend for some depth. The young shoots can be eaten, after blanching in hot water, like asparagus, either steamed or roasted; they can also be pickled. Another old recipe sees the roots being mashed up with cream and salt, rather as you'd do with potatoes. The flesh tastes a bit like carrots, sweeter than you might expect

An easier recipe, which worked well for me, however, is the following and worth trying if only to ask your friends to guess what it is. It is adapted from an Elizabethan recipe and is mentioned in Shakespeare's *Merry Wives of Windsor* as 'snow eryngoes'. The roots of the sea holly extend a long way underground so they are easy to harvest. They're long, brown and stick-like with junctions that give them a bamboo-like appearance. The measurements here can be doubled to make a larger quantity.

Candied Sea Holly

Makes approx 130g

150g eryngo roots, washed and cut into 3cm batons
150g granulated white sugar

Place the roots in a pan and add water to cover the roots by 2cm. Simmer for 10 minutes before adding the sugar. Cook until the sugar has dissolved, then simmer, uncovered, for a further 5 minutes. Leave to stand overnight, making sure that the roots are covered by the cooking liquid – add a little more water if necessary.

Strain the liquid into a clean pan and simmer for 5 minutes to reduce slightly. Add the roots and cook for a further 5 minutes. Remove from the heat and leave to stand overnight again. Repeat the process twice more.

Place the roots on a sheet of greaseproof paper to dry. As they dry, the sugar will crystallise in satisfying lumps on the surface of the roots. They do look a little strange but taste deliciously sweet; you might want to disguise their curious appearance by chopping them up and stirring into Greek yoghurt.

Sedum

Sedum spectabile

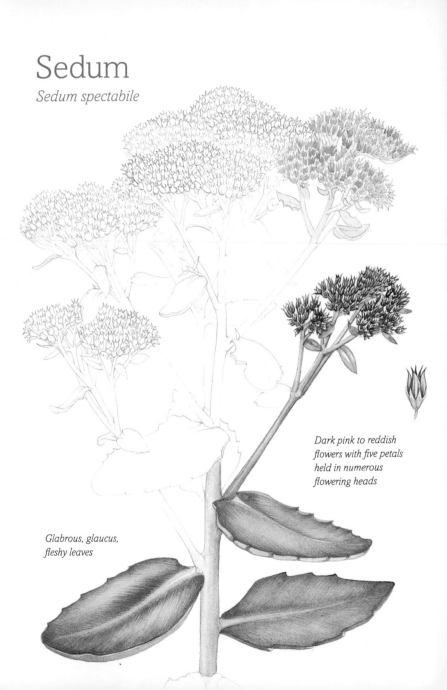

Dark pink to reddish flowers with five petals held in numerous flowering heads

Glabrous, glaucus, fleshy leaves

Sedum belong to *Crassulaceae* family, which are almost exclusively succulents with plump, fleshy leaves and stems which retain water, making them particularly drought resistant.

Succulents, which include cacti and houseleeks, for example, come in a vast range of sizes and colours and it's not surprising that some people make collections of them. Sedum may be annuals or herbaceous or evergreen perennials with succulent stems and leaves and clusters of small, star-shaped flowers in summer or autumn. The flowers of *Sedum spectabile* 'Autumn Joy', illustrated here, open from greenish-pink buds, rapidly progressing through pale pink to become deep pink and ultimately taking on a brownish hue.

Sedum are beautiful plants which thrive with virtual neglect and provide striking colour where many other plants fear to venture. They make themselves at home in the most unpromising of habitats, in the cracks of garden walls or path, make excellent ground cover on otherwise bare and stony ground but also strive in rock gardens, borders and containers. And because of their hardiness and water-retentive characteristics are often used as covering for living or 'green' roof systems. Used in this way, sedums provide a low-maintenance, relatively cheap roof-cover, sold in pre-prepared mats that are rolled out in exactly the same way as turf. An added advantage to using succulents as roofing material is the benefit to birds and insects. (The Rolls Royce car plant in Sussex has an impressive 22,500 square metres of roof, covered entirely in sedums.)

Common Names and Species
Stonecrop, ice plant, orpine, bitter cress, creeping Tom (*S. acre*), rabbit's cabbage.

Medicinal Use
Sedum leaves quench thirst, detoxify and can be used externally to reduce boils and abscesses. An infusion of the leaves of the orpine stonecrop (*S. telephium*) has been a popular remedy for diarrhoea in many countries for centuries.

Culinary Use
All sedums are edible but those with yellow flowers tend towards an unacceptable bitterness. Otherwise, in terms of taste, sedum leaves vary from pleasantly acidic to peppery. One particular variety, the spreading stonecrop (*S. divergens*) was favoured by the Haida peoples of North America as a salad vegetable.

These plants are at their best eaten raw. Their succulent, yet crunchy texture isn't dissimilar to that of cucumber. Houseleeks can be eaten and prepared in the same way.

Sedum Maki Sushi

Sushi is easier to make than you might think and even if the rolling goes wrong, it will taste delicious. You'll need a bamboo rolling mat and these are available in most super-markets, as are the other specialist ingredients.

Makes 24 rolls

140g sushi rice, cooked and cooled
2 tablespoons sugar
2 tablespoons salt
3 tablespoons rice vinegar
3 toasted nori sheets
100g sedum leaves, washed and
  chopped into strips
½ red pepper, finely chopped
¼ ripe avocado, chopped
1 small carrot, grated

First, cook the sushi rice. The tradi-tional way of knowing how much water to add to the rice is to put the rice in the pan, then put your hand into the pan, fingertips on the bot-tom. Add enough cold water to just cover rice. Cook until simmering point, then turn off the heat, cover the pan and leave for 20 minutes. Using this method, you won't need to drain the rice.

In a small bowl, mix the sugar and salt with the vinegar and stir until dissolved. Add to the cooled sushi rice and stir to combine evenly.

Lay out the rolling mat and have a bowl of water and some kitchen pa-per to hand (for wiping your hands).

Place the first sheet of nori on the rolling mat, glossy-side down. Spread some of the rice as evenly as you can on the lower third of the sheet and press it down so that you have a 5mm layer of rice; this takes practice.

Place a line of vegetables – the larger vegetables first and the grated carrot last – across the centre of the rice, pressing them down. Don't overfill the rolls. To roll, take the end of the bamboo mat that's closest to you and fold it carefully over the in-gredients, making sure the bamboo doesn't end up in the filling! Using your fingers, moisten the furthest end of the nori with water. Fold the roll towards the moistened end and seal; squeeze gently and roll the whole thing back and forth across the mat to give it a good cylindrical shape. Slice the prepared nori roll into eight small maki with a very sharp knife. Repeat the whole process with the other two sheets of nori and the re-maining rice and vegetables.

Serve with soy sauce and wasabi.

Instant Sedum 'Pickle'

For this dish, use only the most perfect, fresh and unbruised sedum leaves of whatever variety you have to hand. You can also use houseleek leaves for this pickle.

Serves 4–6 as a side dish

200g fresh young sedum leaves
1 fresh chilli, deseeded and finely
chopped
1 small carrot, washed, peeled and
thinly sliced
2 spring onions, cut into diagonal slices
a small handful of coriander leaves,
torn
½ tablespoon sesame oil
a sprinkle of roasted sunflower seeds
1 teaspoon sea salt

Wash the sedum leaves. Leave whole if they are small and chop larger leaves into evenly sized pieces.

Mix all the ingredients together in a bowl and leave to marinate at room temperature for an hour or so. This is delicious stirred into quinoa.

Spice Bush

Lindera benzoin

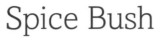

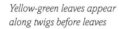

*Yellow-green leaves appear
along twigs before leaves*

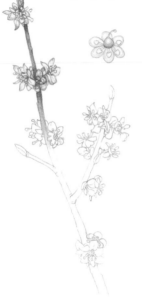

*Highly-polished, scarlet berries
age and dry to a wrinkled brown*

*Glabrous, bluntly oval,
highly-scented leaves*

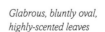

There are several different varieties of *Lindera*, which belongs to the laurel family, *Lauraceae*. This family also includes the bay and the cinnamon plants. The *L. benzoin* variety is the plant we are concerned with here. It's deciduous, can grow to a height of 3m and reaches the same size in width. Although lindera originates from the south-eastern part of Canada and the east coast of the US, it is becoming more popular in the UK and fares well in the northern European climate. The spice bush thrives in partial shade and a neutral soil but prefers slightly acid and wet conditions; the edges of woodlands provide a good habitat. The bushes will grow at altitudes of up to 1,200m.

The pretty, tiny, lemon-scented clusters of yellow flowers – which look as though they've been scattered by hand across the stems and make the bush stand out before the leaves appear – start to bloom in spring, attracting a large range of different insects including the spicebush swallowtail butterfly, which is named after the plant it feeds on. The red, olive-sized berries (the edible part of the plant) start to ripen in late summer.

Common Names

Benjamin bush, fever bush, Appalachian allspice.

Medicinal Use

The name fever bush gives a good clue as to one of lindera's medicinal uses; not, in this case, because the plant stops a fever, but because a tisane of the twigs is used to make the patient sweat profusely, hopefully with the result of alleviating a high temperature; what our grandmothers used to call 'sweating it out'. This is one of the remedies that Native Americans would have used. Once, the bark of *L. benzoin* was used to treat typhoid.

Culinary Use

During the American Civil War the European settlers used spice bush as a substitute when allspice from the West Indies was in short supply.

Break off a twig of the spice bush and you'll release a beautiful, aromatic spicy citrus scent. The berries of the spicebush tree do taste very much like allspice, with echoes of red and black peppercorns with a good smack of cinnamon. It's one of those flavours that is hard to describe because it's so unique and if you have a bush in the vicinity you'll want to harvest as many as you can. You can use them fresh – simply crush both the fruit and the large stone in the middle with a pestle and mortar. You can also freeze the berries. Drying the berries doesn't work, alas, since they're oily and tend to go a bit smelly.

Spice-Bush Ice-Cream

Serves 4

500ml double cream
2 tablespoons honey
a pinch of salt
460ml whole milk
1 teaspoon ground spice-bush berries,
  washed
2 teaspoons vanilla extract

Put half the cream, the honey and the salt into a heavy-bottomed pan. Cook over a low heat, stirring, to melt the honey and then bring to a simmer. Remove from the heat. Stir in the rest of the cream with the milk, ground spice-bush berries and the vanilla. Leave to cool, then cover and refrigerate overnight.

Then either churn the ice-cream in an ice-cream maker, following the manufacturer's instructions, or pour the mixture into a tub and freeze for 1 hour, stir with a fork and freeze again. Leave to stand for 5 minutes before breaking up with a fork once more before serving.

Spice-Bush Chai

Makes 1 cupful

1 mugful full-fat milk
10 fresh spice-bush leaves, washed,
  or 5 dried leaves
sugar or honey, to taste

Put all the ingredients into a heavy-bottomed pan (with a lid) and bring slowly to a simmer, stirring from time to time. Boil for 3–5 minutes, then remove the pan from the heat and cover. Leave to infuse for 10 minutes, then strain the tea to remove the leaves before serving.

Apple and Spice-Bush Chutney

Because apples and spice-bush berries appear at the same time and because this unusual chutney takes 3 months to mature, it's worth making lots of jars to give as Christmas presents.

Makes enough to fill 2 x 450g jars

225g red onions, chopped
900g apples, cored and roughly
  chopped
340g brown sugar
425ml malt vinegar
I garlic clove, roughly chopped
110g dried fruit of your choice (raisins
  are good)
4 teaspoons ground spice-bush berries
  (including the stones)

Place all the ingredients into a large, heavy-bottomed pan and heat gently to dissolve the sugar. Simmer over a low heat for about 2 hours, stirring occasionally so the chutney doesn't catch on the bottom of the pan.

When the surface of the chutney is thick enough to leave a groove when you draw a wooden spoon across it, it's cooked. Spoon into warm, sterilised jars. Leave to cool before putting on the lids. Leave the flavours to mature for 3 months before using.

This is lovely served with a mild, creamy cheese such as Brie.

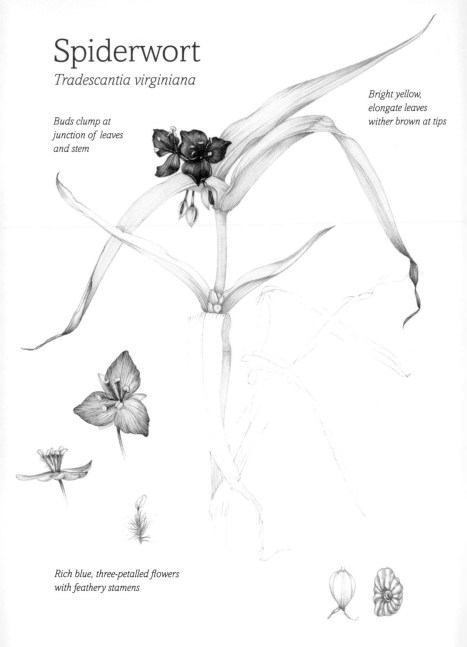

Spiderwort
Tradescantia virginiana

Bright yellow,
elongate leaves
wither brown at tips

Buds clump at
junction of leaves
and stem

Rich blue, three-petalled flowers
with feathery stamens

Tradescantia is named after John Tradescant, one of the earliest English naturalists and a renowned 16th- and 17th-century plant collector who became closely associated with the plant. It is commonly known as spiderwort, because of the long, strappy tendrils like giant spidery legs that dangle down from underneath the flower head.

There are about 70 varieties of tradescantia, which originated in the Americas as a wildflower. It's been a popular garden flower in the UK for almost 400 years now. Where it seeds itself naturally it is generally welcomed rather than weeded out. One variety is a popular pot plant – so popular that I reckon most people have had one at some point in their lives – with stripy, green and purple leaves, known as wandering Jew, purple wandering Jew or, most commonly, spider plant; the tendrils do have a spidery look to them. They make a good pot plant because they're not fussy about where they grow and have a reputation for being virtually impossible to kill. But, if you plan to eat tradescantia, avoid the pot-plant variety because it can sometimes cause a slight irritation to the skin and the inside of the mouth. Try the *fluminensis* or *virginiana* varieties, which both grow prolifically, although the leaves will need to be eaten soon after picking since they darken and go limp after a few hours. These varieties grow in clusters which reach between 30 and 60cm in height, are delicate-looking rather than robust, with long, strappy leaves not unlike those of bluebells, although somewhat thinner and coarser. Likewise, the seed heads, which form after the flowers, look very like those of bluebells. The colours of the flowers range from white through to purple (although most commonly they're a violet-blue), have three petals and twice that number of anthers projecting from the centre of the bloom. Because of the triangular formation of three petals, the flowers look as though they have a little face, a bit like a pansy.

The flowering season for tradescantia is generous, from early summer through to early autumn and even beyond that if the climate is mild enough. They prefer an acidic soil so long as it's on the nutritious side. The plant doesn't mind having its roots in either dry soil or moist (but not waterlogged) and prefers semi-shade. The fringes of woodlands are a good environment for tradescantia. They're easy to grow, requiring little or no maintenance apart from the control of clumps in a limited space. And bees and butterflies love them.

Medicinal Use

Native American tribes had several uses for tradescantia. A poultice was used to soothe insect bites and stings and an infusion of the roots was used for its laxative effect. More unusually, the dried flowers, ground to a powder, were used as a sort of snuff to prevent nosebleeds.

Culinary Use

Tradescantia flowers are a pretty and edible garnish and can be candied too; brush them with beaten egg white, sprinkle with caster sugar and leave overnight to dry. The abundant leaves can be treated like spinach: cook by steaming or sautéing in a little butter or olive oil, then dish up with a hot oil dressing and a little lemon juice and chilli for a delicious side dish. The leaves have a pleasingly mild taste and a cooling effect which complements spicy dishes very nicely. They're also delicious braised in garlic and white wine; if you have the end of a bottle in the fridge this would be the perfect use for it. The seeds, too, are edible; Native Americans toasted them and then ground them into a powder.

Frittata with Tradescantia Leaves and Flowers

Serves 4

2 tablespoons olive oil
400g new potatoes, cooked and roughly sliced (leftovers are fine)
4 eggs, beaten
a handful of tradescantia leaves, washed and ripped into little pieces
5 spring onions, thinly sliced on the diagonal
a handful of chives, chopped
30g strong Cheddar, grated
4 tradescantia flowers, to garnish

Heat the oil in a small, preferably non-stick, frying pan. Fry the sliced potatoes until crisp and golden.

Whisk together all the other ingredients (except the cheese and flowers) and pour over the potatoes, shaking the pan and stirring gently so that the mixture covers the base of the pan evenly.

Cook the frittata over a medium heat for 8–10 minutes. Remove from the heat, then sprinkle the cheese over the frittata and place under a preheated grill to melt and brown the cheese. Use a spatula to loosen the frittata and remove to a warmed plate. Leave to cool for a couple of minutes, then cut into four pieces. Garnish with the tradescantia flowers and serve with a crisp green salad.

Strawberry Tree

Arbutus unedo

Clusters of greenish, pink-tinged, bell-shaped flowers with green anthers

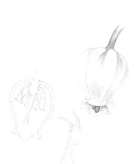

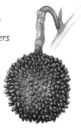

Shiny, oval, slightly serrated leaves

Edible fruit, with orange-yellow flesh, covered in soft spines; starts green, turning yellow, orange to crimson-red when ripe

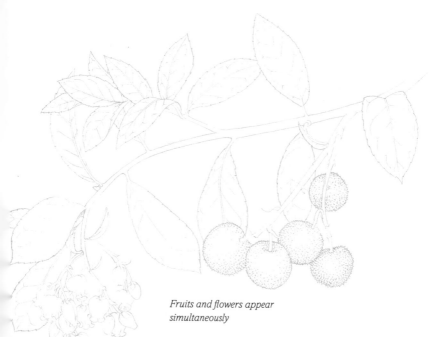

Fruits and flowers appear simultaneously

This plant may be indigenous to Mediterranean areas, but, as some of its names suggest, it has been growing in Ireland for a very long time, particularly in Cork, Sligo and Kerry. There's speculation that it has been there since before the Ice Age and evidence of pollen found in peat bogs indicates that the plant has been a part of the landscape for at least 4,000 years. The Gallic name is *Caithne* and the bay, Ard na Caithne (aka Smerwick), in County Kerry, is named after the arbutus tree. So entrenched is the Irish strawberry there, despite the lack of Mediterranean conditions, that there's even an old traditional poem about it, 'My Love's An Arbutus'. Moreover, it's believed to be the only tree that is effectively native to Ireland but not to the rest of Britain, although the arbutus tree is so beautiful that it is a popular choice in gardens all over the UK as well as in the rest of Europe and America. The Salish tribe of the Pacific Northwest holds the tree in great esteem and never uses the tree as firewood. In their account of the legend of the Great Flood, it was the arbutus to which the Salish tied their canoes to stop them floating away.

Arbutus is a dense, evergreen shrub, growing to some 8m high. Belonging to the *Ericaceae* family, the same as heathers, the arbutus prefers the same growing conditions: acidic soil often found at the edges of woodland and in coastal areas. They don't mind rocky ground or relatively poor soil so long as the ground will hold water and the young plants are protected from harsh winds. The leaves are dark green, quite glossy, approximately 2.5cm across at the widest part with little serrations along the edges. The small blossoms are like a slightly larger version of bell heather, ranging from white to pale pink, borne in clusters and with a slight scent of honey. The flowers and fruits appear in the autumn months and last well into winter. They do indeed look like strawberries, plump and circular, starting life as a pale yellowish-green colour before turning orange and, later, bright red. These fruits are up to 2.5cm across with a rough exterior (think of the surface of a lychee) and apricot-coloured, mealy-textured flesh. The tree bears both blossoms and fruits at the same time, but the berry takes a full year to mature on the branch and is said to be ripe once it drops to the ground. Some gardeners make sure there's a dense layer of grass underneath so the fruits don't bruise when they fall.

Common Names and Species

Irish strawberry, Killarney strawberry, cane apple, bear berry, madrone (*A. menziesii*), Grecian strawberry (*A. andrachne*).

Medicinal Use

The bark and leaves of arbutus are used by herbalists to treat infections of the urinary tract. A gargle of the leaves soothes sore throats. In addition, the astringent bark and leaves were once used as a post-childbirth contraceptive.

Culinary Use

Arbutus means 'struggle' and *unedo* means 'I only eat one'. Now, this could have two opposing meanings: either the fruit is so horrid that you'd only ever eat one of them, or it is so tasty that one is enough. If in doubt, look to tradition; people who have been using the fruits for years advise not to eat them until they have dropped from the trees, when they are at their sweetest and best. Also, until they have dropped there can be very little to distinguish the ripe fruits from the unripe. I'm certain that any misunderstanding about the validity of this fruit is because people might have tried it before it was ready to be eaten. The texture of the inner part of the ripe fruit is quite exotic, a slightly gritty-textured floral flavour not unlike kiwi fruit with a hint of lychee. And sweet, like honey. Also, the reddest fruits are not necessarily the ripest. After the fruit drops but before it goes rotten, the sugars turn to alcohol; if you eat them at this point you'll have a stomach ache and a fuzzy feeling in your head. The Portuguese, Greek and Spanish have worked out how to use these berries to their advantage; they simply add them to brandy to make a ferocious liqueur called *Medronho* in Portugal, *Madroño* in Spain and *Koumaria* in Greece.

Strawberry-Tree Jam

Makes enough to fill 2 x 450g jars

1kg ripe arbutus fruit, picked over
*   and rinsed*
water, to cover
500g golden caster sugar
1 tablespoon orange juice
½ teaspoon vanilla extract

Put the fruit in a heavy-bottomed pan and crush it lightly with a potato masher. Just cover with water, bring to the boil and simmer until the fruit has softened.

Pass the fruit and cooking liquid through a fine-meshed sieve. Discard the pulp and return the strained purée to the pan along with the sugar and orange juice. Cook over a low heat to dissolve the sugar and then turn up the heat. Bring to a rolling boil and cook for 15 minutes, or until a drop of the mixture on a cold saucer wrinkles when you push it with your finger. Stir in the vanilla extract.

Pour into warm, sterilised jars, leave to cool, then seal with waxed discs and put on the lids.

Koumaria Liqueur

If you've been to Greece, you may have noticed hotels and restaurants called Koumaria. There are also several towns and villages of the same name. They are named after the Greek word for the arbutus fruit, *koumara*. The fruit works nicely in a liqueur, and is a very good way of using a minimum amount of fruit to maximum effect.

Note: *You'll need a glass or china container to macerate the fruit; a large-sized rumtopf jar is perfect.*

Makes 1.5 litres

250ml water
500g sugar
250–300g arbutus fruits
70cl bottle of brandy

Pour the water into a heavy-bottomed pan, add the sugar and bring to the boil. Boil for about 5 minutes, or until the sugar has dissolved, to make a syrup. Leave to cool.

Rinse the fruit, then put in a clean jar along with the brandy and pour the syrup over it. Seal the jar, and leave in a dark place for 6 months. After 6 months, strain the alcohol from the fruit. The fruit itself, soaked in brandy, can be used in fruit pies or crumbles or simply eaten with cream.

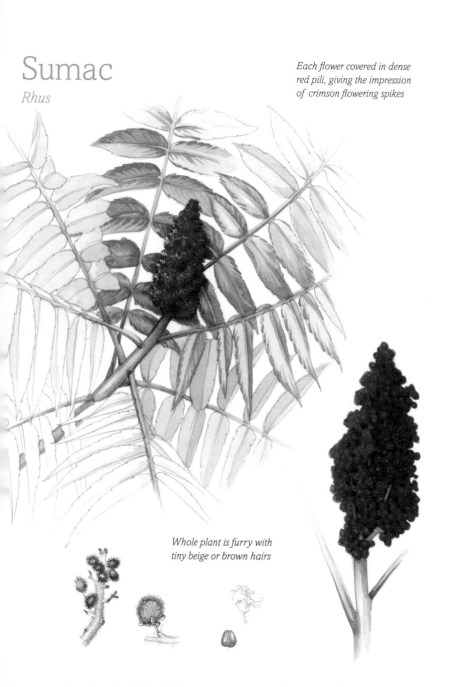

Sumac

Rhus

Each flower covered in dense red pili, giving the impression of crimson flowering spikes

Whole plant is furry with tiny beige or brown hairs

The sumac is an elegant, architectural woody plant whose long oval leaves have serrated edges, radiating out from its curious conical tufts in a five-pointed star formation. Left to their own devices, sumac trees will grow to a height of about 10m. I've seen them growing in industrial estates outside Merthyr Tydfil as well as in large galvanised tubs in a designer roof-garden in Paris, and in both places the plant was thriving.

Originating in the Middle East, across the Mediterranean and in Africa and America, the plant has naturalised in some places to the point of attaining a weed-like status. The tree can be invasive, throwing out suckers and colonising spaces rapidly, and is sometimes treated with disdain, despite its beauty.

There's a sumac, it seems, for all purposes. The reddish-coloured leather bags and souvenirs that you find in Moroccan souks may well be coloured with the *Rhus coriaria* variety (aka tanner's sumac), whereas *R. verniciflua* (Japanese lacquer tree) was at one time used in Japan to make candles. The variety illustrated here and which we tend to see most in ornamental gardens and also as a stray plant is the stag's horn sumac (*R. typhina*). This is so-called because the soft, fuzzy, velvety surface of the tuft resembles the downy texture of a stag's horn.

Common Names and Species

Lemonade tree, stag's horn sumac (*R. typhina*), tanner's sumac (*R. coriaria*), Japanese laquer tree (*R. verniciflua*).

Medicinal Use

As a folk remedy, the bark of the sumac has been used to treat certain STDs as well as diarrhoea. It is also used as a tonic for the bladder and kidneys and can get rid of ringworm.

Culinary Use

Although from a distance they look like flowers, the sumac's upright, gravity-defying, cone-shaped tufts, known as 'bobs', are artfully composed of lots of little fruits of a browny-red colour, each with a fuzzy outer skin and with a solid little seed in the centre. These little fruits are drupes, a fruit with a seed inside; think of the sumac's bob in the same way as a blackberry; a cluster of individual bobbles, each with a pip. The tuft itself will survive the winter in many areas, but the colour does fade in time. Pick the bobs when they're fresh, dark red in colour and during a dry spell; wet weather will wash away the tart, delicious lemon flavour. Simply lick your finger, press it to the side of the bob and lick to check the taste.

Sumac Spice

In the Middle East, for hundreds if not thousands of years, the small seeds inside the drupes have been dried and ground into a mild, lemony-flavoured spice that's almost as ubiquitous as salt and pepper is elsewhere. Until relatively recently it's fair to say that the sumac spice has been the province of the seasoned chef or cook, but it is gradually spreading from the shelves of specialist supplies into more mainstream supermarkets. Or make your own, it's very easy and there's a plant in a garden somewhere nearby. Simply collect 3–4 bobs and leave in a warm, well-ventilated place until completely dry. Break the berries from the bob, pop into a food processor and blitz, in short bursts. Sieve the resulting powder to remove any hard bits, then blitz again until you have a medium/fine powder.

Salmon Sumac Rub

This recipe makes a rather sharp rub that works perfectly with salmon. Add a little brown sugar to sweeten it, or if you like it really sharp, add a little lemon juice with the oil.

Makes about 30g

1 heaped dessertspoon smoked paprika
1 teaspoon sumac berries
1 teaspoon sesame seeds
1 teaspoon Halen Môn celery salt
1 teaspoon dill weed
1 teaspoon white caster or brown sugar
1 teaspoon dried tarragon
½ teaspoon yellow mustard seeds
black pepper, to taste

Using a pestle and mortar or spice grinder, combine all the ingredients and grind to a powder. Don't worry if the sesame seeds stay whole.

For four portions of salmon, mix 1 dessertspoonful of the spice powder with 1 tablespoon of olive or rapeseed oil and rub it over the salmon before roasting, grilling or cooking on a barbecue.

Sumac Lemonade

In North America they call this Indian lemonade or rhus-ade. It is important to use sumac bobs with a good, strong flavour for this recipe. Pick them during a dry spell and check each bob for sharpness and flavour. Never wash the bobs, since you will wash away the flavour.

Makes 1 litre

3–4 sumac bobs
1 litre cold water

Snap each little fruit from the stem into a bowl. Pour the cold water over the top, then mash with your hands or with a potato masher and leave for 6–8 hours before straining into a jug through a fine-meshed sieve or muslin. For a sweeter drink, dissolve sugar to taste in boiling water and add the syrup to the jug.

Fattoush

This is a Levantine bread salad, which uses sumac as a key ingredient.

Serves 4–6

For the dressing
100ml good-quality olive oil
zest and juice of 1 unwaxed lemon
1 small garlic clove, crushed
2 tablespoons sumac spice, made
    as described on page 201
salt and pepper, to taste

For the salad
8 ripe plum tomatoes, quartered
    and deseeded
½ cucumber, peeled and sliced
    into 5cm sticks
½ green pepper, cut into sticks
6 radishes, thinly sliced
1 shallot, thinly sliced
a handful of parsley
a handful of rocket leaves
a handful of mint

To make the dressing, simply whisk all the ingredients together.

To make the salad, toss all the ingredients together in a serving bowl with the dressing. Leave for 15 minutes at room temperature for the flavours to develop before serving. Serve with white pitta bread, torn into little pieces.

Sunflower

Helianthus annuus

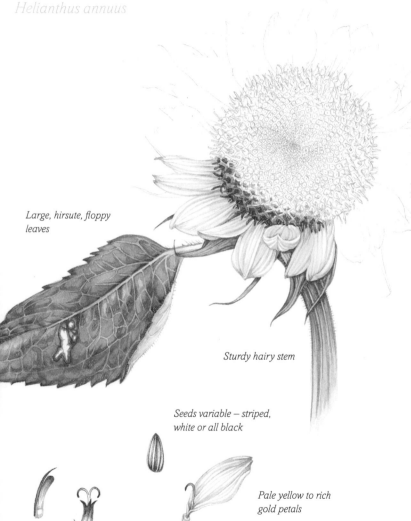

Large, hirsute, floppy
leaves

Sturdy hairy stem

Seeds variable – striped,
white or all black

Pale yellow to rich
gold petals

If sunflowers had the clovey scent of night-scented stock, then it would probably be my favourite flower. The Native Americans first cultivated the sunflower more than 3,000 years ago. Black, blue, purple and red dyes can be extracted from sunflowers; this was a discovery of the Hopi Indians, who also used the tough, fibrous stems and leaves of the plant as material for weaving fabrics and baskets. They also used the oils of the plant to treat insect and even snake bites. The pith of a sunflower stem is even lighter than cork and was once used in the manufacture of buoyancy devices such as lifebelts. The seeds made their way from the Americas to Spain and then to Russia, where it was the first plant oil to be exploited and in the 1950s the very large flowers that we know and love were first bred.

Medicinal Use

At one time, the toasted seeds of sunflowers were ground into an oil which was believed to cure whooping cough. In Turkey, the seeds were made into a tincture and used to reduce fevers in much the same way as quinine. A rather messy-sounding remedy, designed to reduce the feverish temperatures of malaria, was employed in Russia: the leaves were spread out on a bed, soaked in milk and then the unhappy patient was wrapped up in the milky leaves until the fever abated. A fresh leaf preparation was made every day until the patient was cured.

Culinary Use

The simplest thing you can do with sunflowers is to roast the seeds in their shells. If you decide to grow the biggest sunflowers in order to harvest the seeds, do stake the plant; the weight of the heads of the really gigantic ones can sometimes snap the stems, so they will need a bit of extra support. As soon as the petals have fallen, cover the seed heads loosely with a fine mesh. In damp conditions, mildew can form on the seed head so, as soon as the seeds are plump and mature, cut off the entire head and bring it indoors to dry.

To remove the seeds, spread a sheet of newspaper on a table and place the flower head on top. Then just rub the seeds to dislodge them.

To dehusk the seeds before roasting, put a handful of seeds in a ziplock bag, make sure there are no air bubbles and seal it. Then use a rolling pin to gently crack the shells. Pour the contents of the entire bag into a bowl of water; the kernels will sink to the bottom, allowing you to skim the husks from the top.

Roasted and Salted Sunflower Seeds

For every 200g of sunflower seeds in their shells, you'll need (approximately, to taste) 2 tablespoons of salt and one scant litre of water.

Preheat the oven to 200°C/gas 6.

Put the sunflower seeds (in their shells), salt and water in a pan and bring to the boil. Reduce the heat and simmer for 15 minutes.

Drain and give the seeds a good shake. Then spread them in a single layer on a lined baking tray and roast on the top rack of the oven for 10 minutes or until crisp and dry. Keep an eye on them to make sure they don't burn.

Sunflower-Seed Hummus

Serves 4

300g sunflower seeds, dehusked
100g tahini (sesame-seed paste)
1 shallot, finely chopped
2 tablespoons olive oil
1 medium carrot, grated
1 spring onion, finely chopped
salt and pepper, to taste
4 tablespoons fresh lemon juice
100ml water

Toast the sunflower seeds in a dry, heavy-bottomed pan over a medium heat, shaking the pan and stirring all the time to ensure that they don't scorch (this will take about 5 minutes). Leave to cool.

When the seeds are cool, put them in a food processor with the rest of the ingredients (except for the lemon juice and water). Blend for 3 minutes, then add the lemon juice and blend again. Add a little water at a time, and continue to blend until the mixture has the desired hummus-like consistency.

Sunflower-Seed and Chocolate-Chip Cookies

Makes about 50 cookies

125g butter, at room temperature, plus
*   extra for greasing*
300g light brown sugar
1 large egg, lightly beaten
1 teaspoon vanilla extract
350g plain flour
1 teaspoon bicarbonate of soda
100g dehusked sunflower seeds, lightly
*   toasted*
100g chocolate chips

Preheat the oven to 180°C/gas 4. Lightly grease four 30 x 20cm baking trays.

Cream together the butter and sugar with a wooden spoon (or use an electric mixer) until pale and fluffy. Stir in the egg and the vanilla and beat until smooth.

Sift together the flour and bicarbonate of soda over the mixture, then add the toasted sunflower seeds and the chocolate chips and stir to form a dough. Do not overwork the dough.

Form the dough into balls – 50 balls will make biscuits about 4cm in diameter. You can make larger cookies if you prefer. Press each ball on to the prepared baking trays to approximately 1cm thick and leave a 5cm gap around each one to allow for spreading.

Bake for 12–15 minutes, in batches if necessary. Keep any uncooked dough in the fridge before baking.

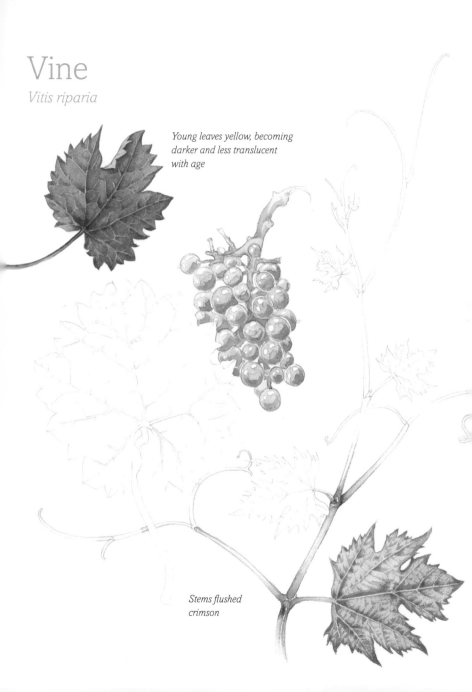

Vine

Vitis riparia

*Young leaves yellow, becoming
darker and less translucent
with age*

*Stems flushed
crimson*

A vine can refer to any plant that uses a structure – a wall, other plants or a man-made framework – to pull itself skywards. Clematis is grouped among the vines, as are morning glory and hops.

But the vine we're interested in here is the ornamental grape vine, *V. riparia*, often grown, not for its fruit, but for its prolific foliage, which turns from a pale fresh green to a rich red towards the end of the summer. There are many cultivars of grape vines, all of which will, under the right circumstances, produce fruit. They like warmth (hence they're often grown under glass) and fertile, well-drained, chalky soil. Vines can grow to a great age – 400 years and over – and very old plants have solid wooden stems which can be cut into planks.

Medicinal Use

Both the leaves and fruit of the vine can be used as a medicine. The fresh leaves were once used as a poultice to cure haemorrhoids, and dried leaves were used to treat dysentery in farm animals. Grapes are traditionally brought to patients in hospitals for very good reason. Grape sugar enters the bloodstream immediately and so is a good source of instant energy.

Culinary Use

Although the grapes from ornamental vines are sometimes so sour as to be inedible, ignored in some cases even by birds, there is still a use for them. Verjuice, for example, is a sour, acidic vinegar made from unripe grapes. It is used in dressings and in cooking whenever a tart flavour is required. You need a lot of grapes to make a little of the juice, though. If you have excess unripe grapes which are unlikely to ripen, collect them together and simply extract the juice, either with a juicer or the old-fashioned way, by mashing and squeezing.

Vine leaves are used all over the world in cooking, perhaps most commonly in *dolmades*, or stuffed vine leaves. Some larger leaves, such as those of the banana, are even used as plates. Vine leaves can be prepared and frozen for convenience. Pick only perfect leaves. Make stacks of the leaves, the biggest at the bottom and the smallest at the top and roll them up. Tie with soft string (so as not to tear the leaves), leaving enough string to dangle over the side of the pan for easy handling.

Then, bring a large pan of salted water to the boil. Using the string, pop the bundles of leaves, one at a time, into the pan. Remove after 15–20 seconds. Drain and leave to cool, then freeze in freezer bags or lidded containers. Defrost the vine leaves completely before using and as the leaves soften by freezing they don't need to be blanched again.

If you want to use fresh leaves, they need to be blanched for 3 minutes before using.

Dolmades

From the Greek word *dolmas*, meaning 'stuffed', *dolmades* are the delicious traditional stuffed vine leaves whose popularity has extended way beyond Greece. If you haven't made them before, don't be daunted by what might seem a complex process. You'll soon get used to placing exactly the right amount of filling on to each leaf.

Pick the tender, fresh leaves at the top of the vine, about the same size as the palm of an adult's hand (approx. 10cm). Smaller leaves are also fine, although they are fiddly to handle. Older, larger leaves tend to be tough but are still useful, so snip off a dozen or so. These will not be eaten, but will be used to line the dish

To prepare the fresh vine leaves, cut off the stem with a sharp knife or kitchen scissors, nicking out the tough end bit that's embedded in the leaf, but take care not to tear the leaf.

For the filling, you can use any combination you like of rice, onions, chopped nuts, raisins, ground meat, herbs and spices. The following recipe works well and makes a nice heap of neat little rolls. The quantities can be halved to make a smaller amount.

Makes 50

50 fresh vine leaves
1 tablespoon vegetable oil, plus extra
for greasing
2 large red onions, very finely chopped
500g Arborio rice, cooked
200g pine nuts, chopped
a handful of herbs (mint, fennel,
chives, basil), finely chopped
juice of 2 lemons
sea salt and freshly ground black
pepper, to taste
olive oil and lemon juice, to serve

Blanch the vine leaves in boiling water for 3 minutes, then place in a shallow dish to cool.

Heat the oil in a frying pan and gently sauté the onions until golden. Stir in the rest of the ingredients, including the salt and pepper, and leave to cool.

Oil a large casserole dish (with a lid), and use the large, tougher leaves to line the bottom of the dish.

Take a vine leaf and place it on a flat surface. Depending on the size of the leaf, place between 1 teaspoonful and 1 tablespoonful of the filling on the leaf – don't be tempted to overfill or the filling will spill out. Fold the pointed bottom of the leaf over the filling, then fold in each side and, finally, roll the top over the whole. Repeat with the rest of the vine leaves, reserving a few larger, tougher leaves.

Carefully place a layer of filled vine leaves in the lined dish close to each other. Cover with the reserved larger, tougher vine leaves. Repeat a final layer of filled vine leaves. Add enough water to just cover the vine leaves, and weight down the leaves with an inverted plate. Cover and cook over a low heat for 1 hour.

Leave to cool to room temperature. Serve with a drizzle of olive oil and lemon juice and a sprinkle of black pepper.

Sharp Grape Jelly

This has a sophisticated flavour and makes a good counterpoint to sweeter meats and cured hams.

Makes enough to fill 2 x 450g jars

1kg grapes
454g white granulated sugar for every
    570ml strained juice (see method)
20g butter

Pick over and wash the grapes and remove the stalks. Put the fruit in a heavy-bottomed pan (with a lid), barely cover with water and bring to the boil. Reduce the heat, cover and simmer for 15–20 minutes or until the grapes are soft. Make sure they don't boil dry, and add a little more water if necessary. Remove from the heat and mash the grapes with a potato masher or the end of a rolling pin.

Strain the grape juice through a jelly bag set over a large bowl or maslin pan and leave to drip overnight.

The next day, measure the volume of juice and weigh out the sugar – for every 570ml of juice you will need 454g sugar.

Put the sugar and liquid back into the pan and, if you have one, clip a sugar thermometer to the inside of the pan. Bring to a rolling boil and heat to 105°C or to setting point. If you don't have a sugar thermometer, use the cold saucer method (see page 13) to test for set. Remove any scum from the surface with a slotted spoon and add the butter right at the end to stop any frothing.

Remove from the heat, leave to cool slightly and pour into warm, sterilised jars. Leave to cool completely, then seal with waxed discs and put on the lids.

Witch Hazel

Hamamelis x *intermedia*

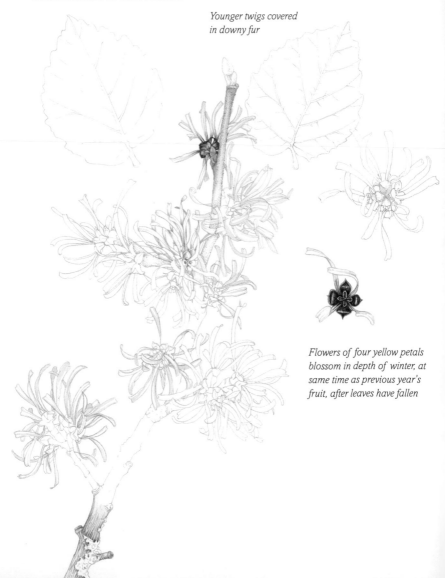

Younger twigs covered
in downy fur

Flowers of four yellow petals
blossom in depth of winter, at
same time as previous year's
fruit, after leaves have fallen

The name of this plant is nothing to do with witches. It is so called because of its supple, bendy branches. The root of the name is in the Middle English word *wiche*, meaning 'pliable', which also gives us the words 'wicker' and 'withy'. Witch hazel's flexible stems are used to make baskets and as divining rods, to detect underground water sources. Native Americans used the wood for making bows. Hamamelis is not particularly edible; however, I wanted to include it here as an example of a garden plant that we regard as being purely ornamental, but which actually has many other uses. Witch hazel has long been used as both a medicine and as a skin cosmetic. It's very easy to make your own witch-hazel remedies at home.

Hamamelis means 'together with fruit'; the flowers and fruits are borne on the branches at the same time. It's a slow-growing shrub, which will reach a height and width of 5m if left unpruned. It will grow in just about any kind of soil so long as its roots are kept damp. Witch hazel was introduced to Europe from North America, although it also grows happily in other parts of the northern hemisphere including Asia. Hamamelis is a perennial, deciduous shrub, with oval leaves. The unusual, spidery yellow flowers appear in the colder months after the leaves have fallen,

growing close to the branches with four long, crinkled petals that look a little bit like lemon peel, not a conventional sort of blossom at all. The seed capsules appear next to the flowers and although there are accounts of the seeds being eaten, for the most part their edibility is debatable, so they're best left alone. If you like winter-flowering plants with a heady, slightly otherworldly scent, then make sure you have witch hazel in your garden. Outdoors, the scent is exotic, very welcome in an otherwise bleak winter landscape. Bring the flowers into a confined space, however, and you'll find they have a distinctly antiseptic, medicinal odour that underpins the medicinal and cosmetic usefulness of the plant itself.

Common Names

Spotted alder, winter bloom, tobacco wood, snapping hazel (due to the loud cracking sounds made by the seeds launching themselves from the seed heads).

Medicinal Use

Native Americans, seemingly, found no end to witch hazel's handiness. As well as a cure for coughs and colds, various tribes used it as an emetic (to cause vomiting), to cure dysentery, to soothe sore eyes, asthma, toothache and cholera and to control haemorrhaging. It was also used to ease bruising of the skin and lesions caused by insect bites. Modern applications of witch hazel by medical herbalists are no less varied and, as well as the applications above, include treating haemorrhoids, as a gargle to soothe throat infections and, possibly its best-known use, as a tonic for the skin. Latter-day herbal practitioners also use witch hazel to ease skin conditions such as eczema and psoriasis, to treat sunburned skin, insect stings and bites, various skin rashes and abrasions, including spots, boils and eruptions, as well as the sorts of injuries associated with childbirth. Witch hazel is astringent and high in tannins, which can help dry, tighten and harden tissues, hence its use in skin applications of all kinds. Additionally, the plant is high in anti-inflammatory and antiseptic properties; among other things this makes witch hazel good to use for sore teeth and gums. Something of a wonder-plant, then!

Witch-Hazel 'Tea'

Makes 1 cup

This tea is an infusion of the leaves and bark, and is very simple to make. You can either drink it or gargle with it, or use it on the skin. Wash a couple of 3–4cm witch-hazel twigs and a leaf, put them in a cup and pour in hot water. Leave to infuse for 5 minutes, then fish out the twigs and leaves with a fork.

Native Americans used this tea to allay the symptoms of colds and flu and, having tried it for the last 4 years, I can report that it seems to be working. The flavour is distinctly 'medicinal' and quite astringent but the addition of some fennel or ginger makes for a more palatable taste. To use on the skin, simply stroke on with a wad of cotton wool and leave to dry naturally. Use as necessary.

Acknowledgments

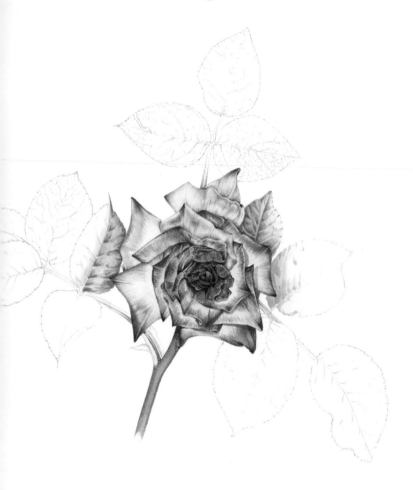

First, I'd like to thank anyone reading this who also bought *The Hedgerow Handbook* (Recipes, Remedies and Rituals). That little book has made me a lot of friends and I am very grateful to all of you.

Thanks to Isabel Atherton at Creative Authors and to James Duffett-Smith.

Thanks are due once again to Rosemary Davidson at Square Peg and the team there who produced this lovely book: Simon Rhodes, Friederike Huber, Rowena Skelton-Wallace, Natalie Wall, Jan Bowmer, Julia Connolly and Ceri Maxwell.

Caroline Danby (www.facebook.com/carolinedanbygardening) provided advice, inspiration and expertise about the plants in this book. David Hardy at the National Botanical Gardens of Wales is a sterling geezer; thanks for your help and support.

I'd also like to thank Carol and Mark at www.foodadventure.com for all their kindness, and also a big shout out to Alexandra, Frank, Tom and Annabel for their 'beyond the call of duty' support (www.alexandramarr.com).

The girls at Brecon Beacons Holiday Cottages, yet again, deserve thanks (www.breconcottages.com).

I'd also like to thank all those who, wittingly or unwittingly, provided plants for me to cook with and for Lizzie to draw. The ones we can mention include The Lovegroves, who provided the splendid *Rosa rugosa*, and Dee Hemmings, who kindly let me plunder her rose garden in search of a different sort of rose; it was hard to know where to start. Donna Darbyshire risked a good drenching to select the finest branches of her sumac, having to balance on a precipitous stepladder right on the edge of the Brecon and Monmouth Canal in a moment that several passing boats will never forget. Alison at The Walled Garden Nursery at Treberfydd (www.walledgardentreberfydd.com) has an amazing variety of plants, as does The Old Railway Line Garden Centre at Three Cocks, near Hay on Wye. And best of all, my lovely old friend Cathy Marchant handily started a cutflower business (Fable Flowers, near Cambridge) just when I needed it, and supplied dahlia roots. If you are one of the people that we scrumped (there were a few), then apologies, but it was all in a good cause and thanks for not calling the police.

Thanks go to my favourite local bookshops and their owners. Buying a book is an experience to be savoured, something which doesn't happen in the same way with online transactions. Hail, Emma at Book-ish in Crickhowell (www.book-ish.com) and Leigh and Nicky at The Hours in Brecon (www.the-hours.co.uk).

And, love and thanks to The Fitzies.

Recipe
Acknowledgments

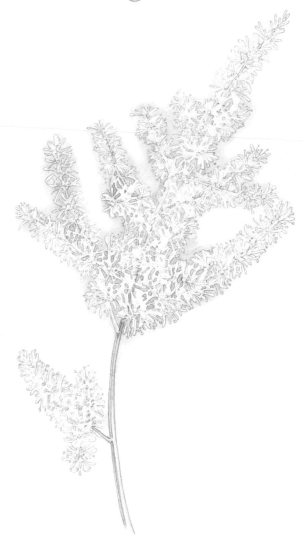

Lots of people contributed specific recipes for this book and others inspired dishes; their details follow.

Denise Baker McLearn, proprietrix of the Moel Faban Supper Club, for the Sumac Salmon Rub recipe (www.moelfabansuppers.com)

Julie Bell and Makthie at the Felin Fach Griffin seemed to crop up whenever anything to do with gin and flowers were concerned and devised the striking Rose Petal Gin recipe (www.eatdrinksleep.com)

www.sweetjamaica.co.uk – Jamaican Calalloo recipe

Maitreya Singh – Keralan Cheera Thoran

Lori Holuta (www.ceelywriter.com) – Juneberry Jelly

Mel and Peter O'Keefe – amelanchier recipes

Liam Fitzpatrick – houttunyia recipes, Sedum Maki Sushi, bamboo-shoot recipes

Yolante Tsiabokalu – Melokhia Soup and Koumaria Liqueur

Jane Preece – Jane's Aronia Layer Cake was devised by Jane Preece

of Burntwood, who raised money for the Teenage Cancer Trust in memory of Stephen Sutton by selling her Aronia Cake samples

Lily Madoc – French Barberry Marmalade

Home Made Country Wines, compiled by Dorothy Wise and published by Countrywise Books in 1955, provided sound instruction for all wine/beer recipes

Sandra Perez (www.tastebook.com) – Chaufa Rice

Spicy Hibiscus Chutney inspired by Miche Bacher's *Cooking with Flowers* (Quirk Books, 2013)

The lovely Lindka Cierach inspired the Lilac Cooler recipe

www.saveur.com – fiddlehead recipes

www.taste.com.au – fish-weed recipes

www.nonabrooklyn.com – Spice-Bush Ice-Cream

www.harvestandyarn.wordpress.com – *cornus kousa* recipes

Pam Corbin inspired the Spicy
Autumn-Olive Ketchup and
Flameberry Pontack recipes

Other online resources that have
wonderful information about the
world of plants and foraging
include www.urbanhuntress.com,
www.punkdomestics.com and
www.thepurpleapple.blogspot.
Greene Deane (www.eattheweeds.
com) hosts the most wonderfully
written and comprehensive blog
about wild edibles that I think I have
ever seen, and Plants for a Future
(www.pfaf.org) is an amazing
organisation and first call to find
out the technical botanical details
of thousands of plants.

Finally, if you would like to contact
me, do so at www.adelenozedar.com

Lizzie is at www.lizzieharper.com

Published by Square Peg 2015

2 4 6 8 10 9 7 5 3 1

First published in Great Britain in 2015 by
Square Peg
Vintage Books, 20 Vauxhall Bridge Road,
London SW1V 2SA

www.vintage-books.co.uk

A Penguin Random House Company

Penguin
Random House
UK

www.penguinrandomhouse.com

A CIP catalogue record for this book
is available from the British Library

ISBN 9780224098892

Penguin Random House supports the Forest
Stewardship Council® (FSC®), the leading
international forest-certification organisation.
Our books carrying the FSC label are printed
on FSC®-certified paper. FSC is the only
forest-certification scheme supported by the
leading environmental organisations, including
Greenpeace. Our paper procurement policy
can be found at www.randomhouse.co.uk/
environment

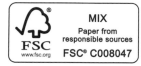

Printed and bound in China by
C&C Offset Printing Co. Ltd